welcome!

During the next five weeks, The 8 Colors program will show you how to approach physical activity in a new way. This innovative program is based on two widely researched and trusted theories: the Myers-Briggs Type Indicator© (MBTI), based on the psychological teachings of Swiss psychiatrist C. G. Jung, and the Stages of Change Model© developed by James Prochaska, PhD, and his research team. The 8 Colors program provides an inspired answer to the question, "What keeps people in a regular exercise program year after year while others drop out?"

This program provides the information, tools, and resources you need to create an exercise program you'll never quit, beginning with the discovery of your unique color-coded fitness personality. As you learn about the natural preferences of your fitness color, you'll find out how to use them to your advantage, choosing the approaches, activities, and environments that are satisfying to you.

You'll also explore the process of self-change and see how to add physical activity at your own pace and with an eye on long-term maintenance of your exercise program. Assessments and exercises reinforce and personalize the program, providing you with a deeper understanding of how you can gain many of the health and wellness benefits of physical activity.

As you work your way through the program, allow time to read each chapter, complete each activity, make notes, and reflect on what you're learning. A page at the end of each chapter is designated for you to keep track of your progress.

You'll learn that change is a process, not a decision, and it follows a predictable course. Understanding your fitness personality will help you keep your unique strengths as an exerciser top of mind and direct you to exercise choices that are the best fit for you. Knowing your fitness personality also helps you identify your unique barriers, which allows you to quickly return to your program in case of backsliding. Let's get started!

Table of Contents

let's get started!

"The secret of getting ahead is getting started."

-MARK TWAIN

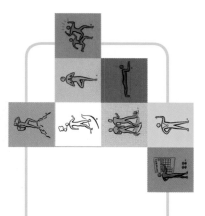
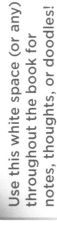

CHAPTER 1

finding your fitness personality

During this first week of The 8 Colors program, you'll learn why the "one-size-fits-all" approach to exercise doesn't work and how it prevents people from maintaining, or even starting, an exercise program. You'll also explore the eight fitness personalities and discover the one that best describes you.

Discover Your Color

To get started, visit www.the8colors.com and click on "take the quiz." Your results will give you a starting place to learn about the factors that will help you become more physically active in a way that is uniquely suited to *you*. And don't worry: If the description doesn't seem like a perfect fit, check page 15 at the end of this chapter for tips on getting a better match.

Before you begin the program:

- Print out the results of the quiz so you can reference them easily.
- Read the first two chapters in The 8 Colors of Fitness (Oakledge Press, 2008) as well as your specific color chapter.
- Read the first chapter of this workbook and complete the activities.
- Take time to reflect at the end by making notes on what you have discovered, and record thoughts or questions you may have.

Use this white space (or any) throughout the book for notes, thoughts, or doodles!

EVERY STEP COUNTS

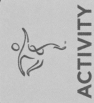

ACTIVITY

How has physical activity decreased in your life?

In a small group or with another person, talk about ways that you (or your parents or grandparents) once included physical activity as part of daily life without thinking much about it. Use the examples as a guide.

Use this white space to complete this exercise.

And don't forget, it's OK for you to write in all the white spaces in this workbook!

IN THE PAST

Walked to school

Took the stairs

Changed television stations manually

Walked, biked, or took public transportation

Shopped on foot

TODAY

Ride the bus

Ride elevators and escalators

Use remote control

Drive or ride in a car

Shop online

With advancing technology, we accept and expect more and more laborsaving devices as a way of life. As our daily lives get easier and more efficient, we take fewer steps and cut back on our physical activity.

How has physical activity been engineered out of your life? Do you remember life before:

- TV remote controls?
- automatic garage door openers?
- "moving walkways" in airports?
- online shopping?

Isn't it amazing how much has changed? Can you see how inactivity has crept up on you? Our way of life naturally used to require more physical activity. Because that has changed — and our need for that physical activity hasn't — we need to move more by making small, intentional changes in daily living.

ACTIVITY

As a first step to a more active life, start thinking about how you can move more throughout your day. Choose a few ways to increase physical activity in your daily life:

Taking the stairs instead of the elevator

Parking in a spot further from your destination

Getting off the bus or train a couple stops early

walking the dog more

PERSONALITY MATTERS

The majority of us have trouble exercising regularly, and while we have many reasons, it often comes down to a lack of enjoyment. It makes sense: When you like what you're doing, you're more likely to keep doing it. If you don't, you won't.

Let's take a look at how your personality and lifestyle have a lot to do with how you'll be successful with regular exercise.

Write your name

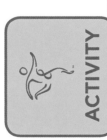

ACTIVITY

In the box below, write your name with your preferred hand. (If you're right handed, write with your right hand; if you're left handed, write with your left hand.)

How did that feel? Most people say writing with their preferred hand feels natural, easy, and comfortable, taking little thought or concentration. Now, in the box below, write your name with your non-preferred hand.

How did that feel? Notice the difference? Most people say writing with their non-preferred hand feels unnatural, difficult, and uncomfortable. The same idea can be applied to physical activity.

Trying to start or stick to an exercise program that doesn't match your personality is like writing with your non-preferred hand. It feels harder, and it takes more energy, so you probably won't stick with it. However, when you're active in a way that matches your personality, you're more likely to have a natural, easy, comfortable experience, like writing with your preferred hand.

THE 8 COLORS OF FITNESS

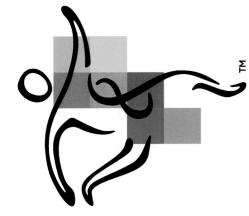

Among other benefits, this program will help you understand your fitness personality so you can create an exercise program that feels natural and that you'll stick with.

This week, you'll learn how the idea of the fitness personality came about.

"What keeps people in an exercise program year after year?" is the question author Suzanne Brue set out to answer.

The potential health consequences of an inactive lifestyle are no secret: heart disease, diabetes, stroke, arthritis, breast cancer, pregnancy complications, infertility, and depression. Nevertheless, a majority of us still have trouble exercising regularly.

Brue saw that the current approach used by fitness experts and medical professionals has some benefits, but it misses a simple truth: Physical activity is an expression of personality, and some activities and environments are more suited to some personality types than others.

Brue, a Myers-Briggs expert, conducted a six-year study in which she interviewed hundreds of physically active people of the 16 personality types according to the MBTI® and gathered self-reported data from hundreds more. She recorded and analyzed the five common factors of exercise for each personality type.

The five factors are: motivation, approach, focus, environment, and interpersonal connections. After evaluating the research, she created a color-coded way to identify patterns based on unique personalities and preferences. That code became The 8 Colors of Fitness (Oakledge Press, 2008).

By identifying your own fitness color and learning more about it, you'll understand why you're drawn to certain activities and environments and why you avoid others. This knowledge will help you make better fitness choices for your personality and take physical activity from boredom to enjoyment.

Let's begin the discovery! On the following pages, you'll find an overview of each of the eight fitness colors. While it's important to read and understand your own, you may also find it interesting to review the other colors and take notice of similarities and differences.

Meet the 8 Colors

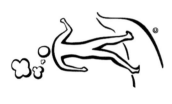

True Blue:
Tried and True

Conscientious, committed, and safety conscious, Blues' approach to exercise is dutiful and without internal debate. They are very tuned in to their bodies, and correct form is essential. Steady and methodical, Blues prefer to focus on one thing at a time. They enjoy keeping track of their progress and take comfort in following programs that have been tested and proven effective.

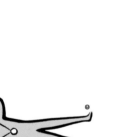

The Gold Standard:
Just the Facts

Traditional and conservative in their approach to exercise, Golds avoid trendy fitness fads. With a reverence for tradition and comforted by the familiar, Golds seek a balanced life, aiming not to overdo. Golds prefer structure and routine, valuing experience, safety, proven methods, and information from experts. They're proud of what they do and enjoy sharing the results.

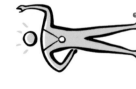

The White Canvas:
Trailblazers on Familiar Paths

Private and self-contained, Whites are attracted to physical activity they can structure at their own pace. Exercise provides alone time for reflection and visioning. Jarred by interruptions and chaos, Whites require orderly environments that provide necessary calm. Outdoor settings and familiar paths and activities are appealing. Advanced planning makes it happen.

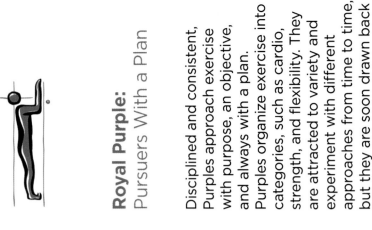

Royal Purple:
Pursuers With a Plan

Disciplined and consistent, Purples approach exercise with purpose, an objective, and always with a plan. Purples organize exercise into categories, such as cardio, strength, and flexibility. They are attracted to variety and experiment with different approaches from time to time, but they are soon drawn back to exercise they can make routine. Once they incorporate exercise into their lives, they generally stay with it.

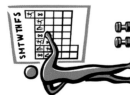

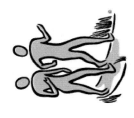

Greener than Green:
Nature Beckons

Minimalist and practical, Greens are naturally observant of the physical details and small variations in their environment. The natural world beckons, and Greens easily blend in. Being outside makes them feel alive, so getting their exercise through activities of daily living, including working outside, makes sense. Greens are motivated to maintain a level of fitness so they can participate in the outdoor activities and challenges that are important to them.

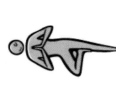

Roaring Reds:
Now!

Fast paced and in the moment, Reds love to be where the action is. Reds experience life through their senses, craving stimulation and adventure from the physical world. Moving is natural; physical activity is about being alive. While Reds are oriented to activity in the physical world, the idea of putting time aside for "exercise" seems tedious and boring unless they are training for a goal with others. Reds understand the importance of fitness and naturally incorporate it in their physically active lifestyle.

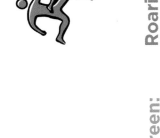

Saffrons Seeking:
Making Workouts into Play

Playful and spontaneous, Saffrons are attracted to activities that are flexible and convenient. Needing opportunities for self-expression, they tend to lose interest in anything too structured. Easily bored and internally demanding of themselves, Saffrons enjoy challenging activities with the right combination of fun, freedom, and flow. A sense of play is appealing, making fun activities, either solo or alongside like-minded others, a high priority.

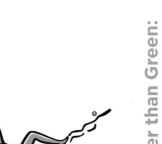

Quicksilver:
Masters of Exercise Disguise

Ingenious and opportunistic, Silvers wrap exercise in a disguise because the idea of pure exercise is unappealing; in fact, having an alternative purpose keeps them engaged in the activity. Silvers enjoy activities that are convenient, requiring minimal process and planning. They are attracted to new ideas and possibilities and to activities that can be done with others. They enjoy variety and tend to cycle through fitness passions. Alternatively, they might avoid the temptation of novelty and keep their exercise program routine and simple.

THE FIVE FACTORS

To more fully understand the concept of the 8 Colors, it's important to be familiar with the five factors that combine to make up each fitness color: motivation, approach, focus, environment, and interpersonal connections. Each personality comprises a different mix of these factors. Understanding your preferences can help you make better decisions about crafting an exercise program that feels most natural, satisfying, and sustainable.

Over the next weeks, we'll take a closer look at each one of these five factors:

FACTOR 1 Motivation

The first of the five factors of fitness personality is motivation: why you exercise, the psychological and emotional points that inspire you and help you maintain an exercise program.

Motivation is the "why?" of your fitness program.

Defining motivation in line with your fitness personality enables you to develop a meaningful workout.

To understand what motivates you, ask yourself:

- What do I personally get out of physical activity?
- What moves me powerfully enough to get over my barriers to exercise?

Examples:

- Blues are motivated by keeping commitments to themselves and accomplishing what they set out to do.
- Silvers are motivated by connections with people and exploring the world.

FACTOR 2 Approach

The second of the five factors of fitness color is approach: how you go about exercise.

Approach is the "how?" of your fitness program.

When you have a successful approach that matches your fitness personality, you're more likely to maintain a consistent exercise program.

To understand your approach, ask yourself:

- Am I more successful approaching exercise as a job and enjoying the sense of accomplishment and order it adds to my day?
- Is a playful approach what gets me to start and stay with a fitness program?

Examples:

- Conscientious Golds prefer exercise to be planned ahead, routine, and structured.
- Playful Saffrons enjoy seizing fitness opportunities, prizing fun and flexibility with limited advanced planning.

FACTOR 3 Focus

The third of the five factors of fitness personality is focus: what engages your mind while exercising.

Focus is the "what?" of your fitness program.

Creating a program that helps you remain engaged will make staying with it much easier.

To understand your focus, ask yourself:

- What do I like to pay attention to?
- What helps me get the mental stimulation necessary to stick with my workout program?

Examples:

- Greens enjoy connecting with what's in front of them, savoring the details and small variations in nature.
- Whites are energized by activities that allow for internal reflection and opportunities to zone out.

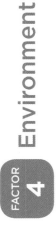

FACTOR 4 Environment

The fourth factor of fitness personality is environment: where you like to exercise, the external factors most likely to support a sustained exercise program.

Environment is the "where?" of your fitness program.

Many environments support activity, and choosing the right one(s) for your fitness personality is the key to keeping your energy up and sticking with an exercise program.

To understand your preference for environment, ask yourself:

- Do I mostly enjoy the outdoors?
- Would I rather go to a fitness center or work out at home?
- Do I like a combination of both?

Examples:

- Purples enjoy the many offerings of a well-organized fitness center.
- Greens recharge their batteries outside.

FACTOR 5 Interpersonal Connections

The fifth factor of fitness personality is interpersonal connections: who you exercise with, your preference for or type of involvement with others while exercising.

Interpersonal connections is the "who?" of your fitness program.

For some fitness colors, working out with others provides fun, momentum, and accountability. For others, working out alone is desirable and energizing.

To understand your preference for interpersonal connections, ask yourself:

- How do I prefer to be involved with others while exercising?
- Does interacting with others keep me going, or does it prevent me from getting the most out of my exercise program?

Examples:

- Blues are internally motivated and prefer routine exercise with minimal interaction with others.
- Reds are stimulated by training with others, and their energy can diminish when they are alone.

Is exercise job or play?

One of the most significant discoveries from Brue's research on fitness personality is the job/play divide. It influences your physical activity preferences in many important ways. In fact, understanding which side of the divide you are on is the single most significant issue in defining your entire approach to exercise. For example, you may have heard that one way to stay committed to your exercise program is to find an exercise buddy, but Brue's research indicates that this is not necessarily true for all personalities. In fact, for some, trying to include others in an exercise program may hurt rather than help.

Job Exercisers

People who approach physical activity from the job perspective usually think of exercise as part of their overall daily or weekly plan. They feel energized by defining and completing their exercise plans. Although they may get enjoyment or satisfaction out of exercise, fun is not the motivator. Instead, motivation often comes from a sense of accomplishment by finishing their plan. Job exercisers don't like being swept into other people's agendas. They don't necessarily avoid having others in their exercise environment, but they prefer to keep their interaction to a minimum and enjoy being with their own thoughts.

Blues, Golds, Whites and Purples are job exercisers

Play Exercisers:

People who approach exercise from the play perspective usually prefer an element of fun, learning, exploration, or connection with others. They have a spontaneous nature and may feel burdened or inhibited by imposed routines, schedules, or plans. Play exercisers often gain energy by turning their attention to the outer world, and they like exercise to be disguised as something else, such as a social interaction, competition, or a way of enjoying the outdoors.

Greens, Reds, Saffrons and Silvers are play exercisers

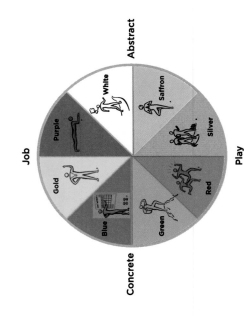

The Color Wheel is a visual illustration of how the fitness colors are related to each other. The job/play and concrete/abstract divides split the wheel. You'll see this color wheel each week throughout the program.

The Concrete/Abstract Divide

Another way to understand the differences between the fitness colors is through the concrete/abstract divide. This division considers the way fitness personalities prefer to notice or gather information while exercising.

Concrete Exercisers:

These personalities naturally notice the physical details around them. They enjoy being outside so they can take in the sights and sounds of nature and the physical environment. They rely on their senses to gather information, such as seeing rough spots on a recreational path, changes in the weather, or new equipment at the fitness center. They are more aware of their bodies and like exercise that enables them to experience their senses and bodies while exercising.

Blues, Golds, Greens, and Reds are concrete exercisers

Abstract Exercisers:

These personalities rely on patterns and abstractions to inform them. They enjoy being outside for the sense of freedom the natural world provides. Their minds are occupied with connections and interpretations, and they may be unaware of their surroundings. They prefer exercise that allows them to be distracted by something else: their inner thoughts, a conversation with another person, music, a spiritual practice, or learning something new.

Whites, Purples, Saffrons, and Silvers are abstract exercisers

Finding the color that fits

Your results on The 8 Colors quiz are a good starting point in identifying your fitness color. Most people feel that their results on the quiz are a good fit. However, some don't. It's not unusual to be unsure about your color the first time you take the quiz.

Here are some suggestions to help you discover your truest fitness color:

- Read the summaries of other colors to see if another description feels like a better fit. In particular, read the descriptions of the fitness colors on either side and across from you on the color wheel (for example, if you are a Blue, read the Gold and Green descriptions as well). All the color summaries can be found online at www.the8colors.com.
- Try taking the quiz again at another time. Your responses can be influenced by how you are feeling at that moment or particular adaptations you might be making at that time.

As you go through this process, keep in mind that discovering your fitness color is not an exact science. Even when the fit is right, it's possible that most items in your color description will sound like you, but a few may not. Some people may feel their color information describes them perfectly while others will eventually choose one that feels *mostly right*.

NOTES

Use this page to reflect on what you've learned, both about The 8 Colors program and about yourself. **Consider the following questions as a guide:**

What is your fitness personality color?

What seems obvious now that you hadn't thought of before?

Where do you fall on the job/play divide? How might that influence your exercise program?

What have you learned this week that might explain why you haven't successfully maintained an exercise program in the past?

Other....

Use this white space for your notes!

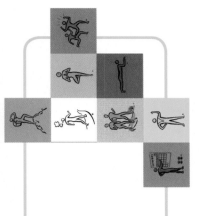

CHAPTER 2

motivation:
why do you exercise?

Welcome to week two! Now that you've discovered your fitness personality, the next step is to identify the five factors of your fitness personality. The first of the five factors of fitness personality is motivation. In addition you will learn about The Stages of Change Model, the benefits of exercise, and the CDC guidelines for exercise.

Don't forget to use the white space!

 FACTOR 1 Motivation

Motivation is the "why?" of your fitness program.

Defining motivation in line with your fitness personality enables you to develop a meaningful workout.

To understand what motivates you, ask yourself:

- What do I personally get out of physical activity?
- What moves me powerfully enough to get over my barriers to exercise?

On the next page, you'll find a review of the physical activity motivators for each of the eight fitness colors. In addition to reading the list for your own color, read the lists for the colors that are next to yours and across from you on the color wheel. Why? You're likely to have a lot in common with those colors and may discover other motivators that you can relate to. For example, if you are a Blue, read the Gold and Green motivators as well. As you read the three lists, circle any phrases that describe you.

Color-Specific Motivators: Why do you exercise?

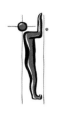

Blue

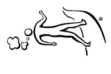

- ○ Keeping commitments I make to myself
- ○ Completing what I set out to do
- ○ Having clear fitness goals
- ○ Following advice from health professionals or trusted sources

Gold

- ○ Keeping commitments to myself and others
- ○ Sharing accomplishments with others
- ○ Having clear fitness goals
- ○ Following advice from health professionals or trusted sources

White

- ○ Enjoying physical activities as a time to reflect and think
- ○ Accomplishing what I set out to do
- ○ Interacting with the outdoors
- ○ Engaging in activities that benefit mind and body

Purple

- ○ Enjoying physical activities as a time to reflect and think
- ○ Accomplishing what I set out to do
- ○ Staying in shape and taking care of myself
- ○ Creating balance in my life

Green

- ○ Reenergizing myself outdoors
- ○ Having fun interacting with the outdoors
- ○ Getting in shape for meaningful outdoor activities
- ○ Increasing my self reliance and preparedness

Red

- ○ Reenergizing myself outdoors
- ○ Having fun interacting with the outdoors
- ○ Enjoying a physically active lifestyle
- ○ Engaging in fun, competitive activities with others

Saffron

- ○ Reducing internal stress and boosting energy
- ○ Finding pleasure in interesting and unusual challenges
- ○ Participating in activities that benefit mind and body
- ○ Seeking enjoyment in the activity, with exercise as an added benefit

Silver

- ○ Responding to threats to health and well-being
- ○ Finding pleasure in exploration and novel experiences
- ○ Participating in activities that benefit mind and body
- ○ Seeking enjoyment in the activity, with exercise as an added benefit

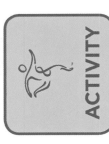

ACTIVITY

Put your preferences into practice

Focusing on ways you can consistently connect with the activities that you personally find meaningful will help you keep your commitment to your fitness routine.

Also important:

- Resist the temptation to follow advice that does not match your personal motivators
- Stop looking for inspiration for exercise in the wrong places
- Use your personal motivators to gain the mental strength and positive experiences you will need to be successful!

The following activity will help you discover how to use your personal motivators effectively. In the left column, choose the fitness color motivator from the previous page that best describes you. Next to the motivator, describe how you'll put it into action.

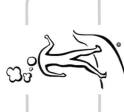

MOTIVATOR

Example from a White:

1. Engaging in activities that benefit mind and body

HOW YOU'LL USE IT

1. Research yoga online — what are the benefits and where should I start?
2. Go to the yoga studio in my neighborhood to check it out and get a class schedule.
3. Use my morning walks as a time to reflect and think.

UNDERSTANDING CHANGE

Change: a process not a decision.

"Just do it!" If only making a behavior change were as easy as the popular Nike slogan makes it sound.

Realistically, starting and sticking with a regular exercise program is achieved not with the snap of a finger or a one-time decision but by cycling through a process that has predictable stages.

The Stages of Change Model® was developed by behavior change researchers James Prochaska, John Norcross, and Carlo DiClemente. Along with other self-change researchers, they studied thousands of successful self-changers and saw that lasting behavior change is a staged process with a predictable pattern. The Stages of Change Model has been studied and tested widely, revised, and improved through "scores of empirical studies" (14). It is currently used by professionals around the world and has revolutionized the science of behavior change.

It is a fundamental part of The 8 Colors program.

The Stages of Change.

Specific to physical activity, you might think about **the stages** as follows:

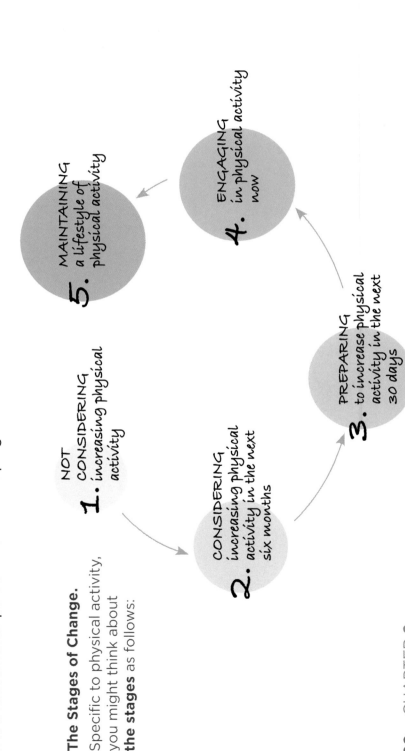

1. NOT CONSIDERING increasing physical activity

2. CONSIDERING increasing physical activity in the next six months

3. PREPARING to increase physical activity in the next 30 days

4. ENGAGING in physical activity now

5. MAINTAINING a lifestyle of physical activity

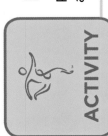

ACTIVITY

Know your stage

Review the following five statements and select the one that best describes you at this moment. Then circle the name of the stage to the right of the statement.

I'm not considering becoming more physically active right now, or I'm considering it but don't think I'm likely to make the change now.

1. NOT CONSIDERING

I'm considering becoming more physically active in the next six months.

2. CONSIDERING

I'm preparing to become more physically active within the next 30 days.

3. PREPARING

I'm presently engaging in physical activity.

4. ENGAGING

I've made physical activity a habit and have been maintaining this habit for six months.

5. MAINTAINING

More about the stages

Below is a brief description of each stage and some recommendations to help you move to the next stage:

1. NOT CONSIDERING

At this stage, you are not currently considering exercise or the benefits of changing. When people are not even thinking about increasing their physical activity, it's usually because they fall into one of two mindsets:

In the "I won't" mindset, individuals are not interested in increasing their physical activity because they don't believe their inactivity is a problem.

In the "I can't" mindset, individuals want to be more active but don't believe it's possible.

At this stage, the cons of changing the status quo outweigh the pros of exercise.

2. CONSIDERING

If you're in the considering stage, you've begun thinking seriously about becoming more physically active. This is the "I may" stage. You are still sitting on the fence, but you are becoming more aware of the benefits of physical activity and are looking at managing some of the barriers that have been holding you back.

At this stage, you might be interested in learning about the strengths of your fitness color.

You are less satisfied with things as they are, beginning to evaluate the pros vs. cons, and considering becoming more active in the next six months.

3. PREPARING

If you're in the preparing stage, you're ready to increase your physical activity in the next 30 days. This is the "I will" stage. Depending on your fitness color, you may be visiting fitness centers, noting recreational paths, talking to your physically active friends, and starting to brainstorm what activities reflect your fitness color.

The pros of becoming more physically active are beginning to outweigh the cons, and you are considering becoming more physically active in the next 30 days.

4. ENGAGING

At this stage you are actively making changes. You're increasing your physical activity and starting to work up to your exercise goals. You've identified activities and environments that match your fitness color.

You're creating realistic action plans and learning to deal with your barriers or setbacks. This is the "I am" stage. The pros have outweighed the cons. You're beginning to experience the benefits of a physically active lifestyle.

5. MAINTAINING

At this stage, you have been physically active for at least six months. This is the "I still am" stage. You've learned to make exercise choices that suit your fitness color and are enjoying the benefits of your physically active lifestyle. You've made the necessary changes in your lifestyle to fit physical activity into your week and have successfully dealt with your color-specific barriers.

You're generally feeling more comfortable and confident that you can make physical activity a habit.

The benefits of exercise

Research has proven that physical activity is an important component of a healthy lifestyle; it improves our overall vitality in just about every way. If knowing that exercise is good for us were enough, the majority of us would be more physically active. Instead, less than 30 percent of the population is active enough to reap the benefits of a physically active lifestyle. In an effort to understand what motivates people to exercise, Brue interviewed successful exercisers of every fitness color. As part of her interview she asked, "Why do you exercise?"

The following are highlights of the color-specific motivators for all the fitness colors. Look at the motivators and add some more of your own.

Exercise helps me to:

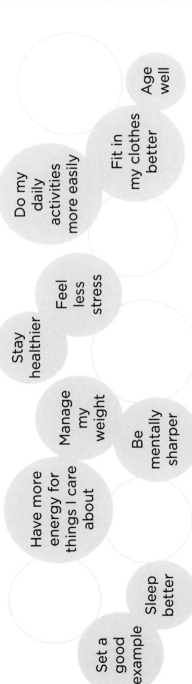

Set a good example

Sleep better

Have more energy for things I care about

Manage my weight

Be mentally sharper

Stay healthier

Feel less stress

Do my daily activities more easily

Fit in my clothes better

Age well

Review your color-specific motivators that you identified on page 18. Look again at the lists next to yours on the color wheel and at the generic motivators above.

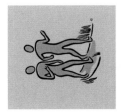

LINDA, A SILVER, WAS AMAZED WHEN SHE LEARNED HOW HER FRIEND JENNIFER, A BLUE, STAYS MOTIVATED FOR EXERCISE:

"I've always admired how my friend Jennifer sticks to exercise so regularly. She's at the gym four days a week like clockwork and she never seems to struggle with the lack of motivation for exercise like I do. She said she just makes a mental commitment to do it and gets it done. I couldn't believe it when she told me that she doesn't always enjoy the exercise while she's doing it but that she gets satisfaction out of having done it. That would never work for me! I really need to have fun while I'm exercising — and I love being with other people while I'm doing it."

ACTIVITY

What motivates you?
Write down the six reasons that are most motivating for you.

With a partner, discuss your top motivators. Give examples of why they are motivating for you.

What motivates you?

1.

2.

3.

4.

5.

6.

Why?

1.

2.

3.

4.

5.

6.

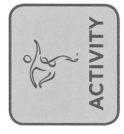

ACTIVITY

Interview someone who gets regular exercise

Think of a friend, family member, or coworker you know who exercises regularly. Ask if he or she would be willing to spend 20 to 30 minutes with you discussing how and why he or she exercises. (People who live physically active lives are often more than happy to talk about them!) Before you do the interview, ask her/him to take the short fitness color quiz. Ideally, your interviewee should be someone who is a different color than you.

Completing this interview will be beneficial because it will help you:

- Learn how others are successful with exercise
- Understand how the five factors (motivation, approach, focus, environment, and interpersonal connections) contribute to their success
- Recognize how others' exercise choices are like and/or unlike yours

Interview Questions

1. What is your fitness color?

2. What do you do for exercise?

3. Why are you motivated to exercise?

Use the white space for
your interview answers!

4. How did you create your fitness program?

If you need more inspiration, review your color's chapter in The 8 Colors of Fitness book.

GET THE BOOK ON AMAZON.COM!

Read the interviews and jot down routines that inspire you.

1.

2.

3.

5. Where do you prefer to exercise? What aspect or aspects of the environment are important to you?

6. Who do you prefer to exercise with — alone or with others? If with others, describe the interactions that you most enjoy.

7. What do you focus on while you are exercising? Do you need something to distract yourself or does your mind wander?

What constitutes "enough" exercise?

Knowing why you are motivated — and why not — is one of the most important considerations in starting and maintaining a more active lifestyle. But what exactly is a "more active lifestyle"? And how much exercise do you need to gain the health benefits we hear so much about? According to research by the Centers for Disease Control and Prevention, an adult needs to accumulate 150 minutes of moderate intensity activity or 75 minutes of vigorous intensity activity (10 minutes at a time is fine!), plus strength training twice weekly hitting the major muscle groups.

http://www.cdc.gov/physicalactivity/everyone/guidelines/adults.html

Definition of Moderate Activity and Vigorous Activity

A MET (Metabolic Equivalent of Task) is the energy cost of physical activities. The chart below will give you an idea of the METs for different activities — ranging from light to moderate to vigorous. For more information on METs, visit:

http://www.cdc.gov/nccdphp/dnpa/physical/pdf/PA_Intensity_table_2_1.pdf

- Activity that burns fewer than 3 METs is considered light intensity activity
- Activity that burns 3-6 METs is considered moderate intensity activity
- Activity that burns more than 6 METs is considered vigorous intensity activity

---

Physical Activity

Light intensity activities < 3 METs

- Sleeping
- Television
- Reading, writing, meditating
- Walking, 1.7 mph, level ground, strolling, very slow

Moderate intensity activities 3-6 METs

- Walking 3 to 4 mph on a level surface
- Cardio machine, e.g., stationary bike, treadmill, Stairmaster
- Bicycling less than 10 mph
- Tennis doubles
- Light yoga

Vigorous intensity activities > 6 METs

- Race walking, jogging or running
- Cardio machine, e.g., stationary bike, treadmill, Stairmaster
- Bicycling more than 10 mph
- Energetic ballroom dancing
- Tennis singles

Meet the Guidelines Your Way

Be true to your color: To successfully increase your level of physical activity, be sure to do so in a way that honors your preferences. The CDC guidelines provides a goal, but how you get there is up to you. Here are eight color-specific examples of different ways to meet the recommended guidelines for physical activity. Remember 10 minutes at a time will get you there!

blue

150 minutes of moderate activity
- Walk briskly walk alone on a familiar outdoor path, measuring time or distance. *3x week (30 min) = 90 min*
- Work out on your favorite cardio machine. Stay engaged watching TV, listening to music, or reading. *2x week (30min) = 60 min*

75 minutes of vigorous activity in a week:
- Run alone on a familiar outdoor path, measuring time or distance. *3x week (25 min) = 75 min*

Strength Training
Attend a trusted group strength training class, hitting all major muscle groups. Same time/same place. *2x week.*

gold

150 minutes of moderate activity
- Walk briskly on a familiar outdoor path, measuring time or distance. Share accomplishments with friends and family. *2x week (25 min) = 50 min*
- Swim laps in a pool, tracking progress. *2x week (25 min) = 50 min*
- Attend a trusted, well-organized group fitness class. *1x week = 50 minutes*

75 minutes of vigorous activity in a week:
- Run on a familiar path. Share your accomplishments. *2x week (15 min) = 30 min*
- Attend indoor cycling class. Choose a qualified instructor with easy-to-follow cuing. *1x week = 45 min*

Strength Training
After instruction from a qualified trainer, use strength-training equipment at a fitness center to work all major muscle groups. Record and keep track of progress. *2x week.*

white

150 minutes of moderate activity
- Walk briskly on a familiar outdoor path, one that is calm and peaceful. *3x week (30 min) = 90 min*
- Ride a stationary bike while reading. Go to fitness center at off-peak times. *2x week (30 min) = 60 min*

75 minutes of vigorous activity in a week:
- Run alone on a familiar outdoor path, calm, peaceful, and away from commerce. *3x week (25 min) = 75 min*

Strength Training
Attend a yoga class that focuses on strength and targets all major muscle groups. *2x week.*

purple

150 minutes of moderate activity
- Walk briskly, generally keeping track of distance or time. *2x week (30 min) = 60 min*
- Bike on a level terrain at speeds 5 to 9 mph. *2x week (30 min) = 60*
- Work out on elliptical machine, while watching TV or listening to music. *1x week (30 min) = 30 min*

75 minutes of vigorous activity in a week:
- Run in a familiar environment. *2x week (25 min) = 50 min*
- Bike on hilly terrain, or at speed more than 10 mph. *1x week (25 min) = 25*

Strength Training
With a personal trainer, design a strength-training program that targets all major muscle groups, and can be done at home or at a fitness center. *2x week.*

green

150 minutes of moderate activity

- Walk briskly outside. Go when the moment or changing weather system invites. *2x week (25 min) = 50 min*
- Increase time on daily activities, e.g., parking further from your destination, taking the stairs, gardening. *5x week (10 min) = 50 min*
- Attend a Pilates or yoga class. *1x week = 50 min*

75 minutes of vigorous activity in a week:

- Use your own body for a full body workout. Include exercises such as push-ups, plank, chin-ups, leg raises, lateral walks, squats, and lunges. *3x week (25 min) = 75 min*

Strength Training

Use your own body for a full body workout. Include exercises such as push-ups, plank, chin-ups, leg raises, lateral walks, squats, and lunges. *2x week.*

red

150 minutes of moderate activity

- Meet up with a friend or a group for a bike ride. *2x week (25 min) = 50 min*
- Meet up with friends for a casual game of basketball or doubles tennis. A post-game get together will make it more fun. *2x week (25 min) = 50 min*
- Attend a group fitness class with great music. *1x week = 50 min*

75 minutes of vigorous activity in a week:

- Train for a half-marathon with a friend or group of friends. Remember, a post-workout get together will make it more fun. *2x week = 60 min*
- Jump rope outside to energetic music. *1x week = 15 min*

Strength Training

Attend an action packed boot camp that targets all muscle groups. *2x week.*

saffron

150 minutes of moderate activity

- Go for a brisk walk alone or with people you enjoy spending time with. *2x week (25 min) = 50 min*
- Attend a cardio-dance class. Flexible scheduling and great music is a plus. *1x week = 50 min*
- Attend a yoga class with agreeable flow and music. *1x week = 50 min*

75 minutes of vigorous activity in a week:

- Meet with people you enjoy spending time with for a run. *1x week = 50 min*
- Jump rope, hula hoop, or jump on a trampoline. *1x week = 25 min*

Strength Training

Use your own body and bands for a full body workout. Include exercises such as push-ups, burpees, chin-ups, leg raises, crunches, tuck jumps, squats, and lunges. *2x week.*

silver

150 minutes of moderate activity

- Meet up with a friend or group for a brisk walk. Confirm by texting prior to walk. *2x week (30 min) = 60 min*
- Bike to a friend's house, visit, then bike home. *1x week = 30 min*
- Attend a cardio fitness class. *1x week = 60 min*

75 minutes of vigorous activity in a week:

- Train for a triathlon with a friend or group of friends. *3x week = 75 min*

Strength Training

Meet a personal trainer at a fitness center for a one-on-one session 1x week, plus, attend a group fitness strength training class. 1x week.

NOTES

Use this page to reflect on what you've learned, both about The 8 Colors program and about yourself.

Consider the following questions as a guide:

What stage of change are you in?

What color-specific motivators most apply to you?

How might you use these motivators in your own life?

What have you learned this week that might explain why you haven't successfully maintained an exercise program in the past?

What do you think of the CDC guidelines?

Other....

Use this white space for your notes!

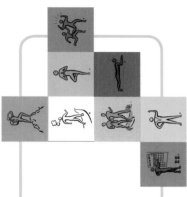

CHAPTER 3

approach and focus:
how do you exercise and engage your mind?

Welcome to week three! Now that you've discovered why you are motivated, the next step is to explore the second and third factors. You'll learn the best ways to set about your fitness program so you'll stick with it and how to choose effective thoughts that support you as you make positive changes. Then, you'll explore the source of your mental energy and what engages your mind while exercising. In addition, you'll have an opportunity to create a 4-day win!

FACTOR 2 Approach

Approach is the "how?" of your fitness program.

When you have a successful approach that matches your fitness personality, you're more likely to maintain a consistent exercise program.

To understand your approach and what keeps you engaged, ask yourself:

- Am I more successful approaching exercise as a job and enjoying the sense of accomplishment and order it adds to my day?
- Is a playful approach what gets me to start and stay with a fitness program?

Examples:

- Playful Saffrons enjoy seizing fitness opportunities, prizing fun and flexibility with limited advanced planning.
- Conscientious Golds prefer exercise to be planned ahead, routine, and structured.

On the next page, you'll find a summary of the preferred approach to physical activity for each of the eight fitness colors. In addition to reading the list for your own color, read the lists for the colors that are next to yours on the color wheel. As you read the three lists, circle any phrases that describe you.

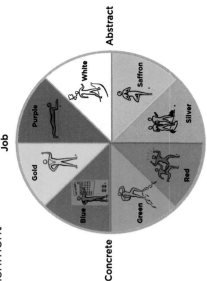

Color-Specific Approaches

Blue

- Planning and scheduling my exercise program in advance
- Being sensible and learning safe and correct exercise form from the start
- Building my program step-by-step and achieving measurable goals along the way
- Choosing activities that I can make part of my routine

Gold

- Planning and scheduling my exercise program in advance
- Being sensible by learning safe and correct exercise form from the start
- Setting long-term goals, then breaking goals into smaller measurable pieces
- Choosing activities that I can make part of my routine

White

- Researching; then building a program based on my self-defined goals
- Planning my exercise program in advance
- Classifying exercise into categories, such as cardio, strength, and flexibility
- Choosing activities that I can make part of my routine

Green

- Keeping gear handy to be ready for action
- Having fun; avoiding joyless exercise
- Staying open to unplanned opportunities
- Getting exercise through activities of daily living

Red

- Keeping gear handy to be ready for action
- Staying open to unplanned physical activity
- Participating in competition with others and enjoying many ways to win
- Having fun with many types of exercise

Saffron

- Seeking activities that are fun, yet challenging
- Having fun; avoiding joyless exercise
- Participating in activities that are personally appealing and often unusual
- Choosing activities that are convenient, requiring minimal process and advanced planning

Purple

- Researching, consulting with experts, then building a program based on my self-defined goals
- Planning my exercise program in advance
- Classifying exercise into categories, such as cardio, strength, and flexibility
- Experimenting occasionally, but staying with activities that I can make routine

Silver

- Participating in activities that hold my attention with several layers of interest
- Having fun; avoiding joyless exercise
- Choosing activities that are convenient, requiring minimal process and advanced planning
- Keeping exercise easy to complete

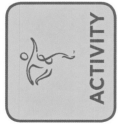

ACTIVITY

Put your preferences into practice

Your preferred approach to exercise is a personal strength that you can use to create strategies and positive experiences. As you work toward a steady physical activity program, it's important to understand and connect with your preferences. Friends, family members, and others may try to help you create your program, but their help may not always match your true fitness color. Be sure to stay focused on the strategies that support your true color.

The following activity will help you discover how to use your personal approach effectively. In the left column, choose the fitness color approach from the previous page that best describes you. Next to the approach, describe how you'll put it into action.

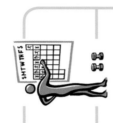

APPROACH

Example from a Blue:

1. Build my program step-by-step, achieving measurable goals along the way

HOW YOU'LL USE IT

1. Talk with other Blues about how they got started exercising

2. Set up an appointment with a personal trainer at my fitness center to develop a workout plan and realistic goals

3. Work on increasing cardio by 3 to 5 minutes each session for now, and add in weights when I am ready.

JANE, A GOLD, DISCOVERED THE IMPORTANCE OF UNDERSTANDING HER OWN AND OTHERS' APPROACHES THIS WAY:

"For months, I've been trying to get my partner to exercise by asking him to commit to walking with me three times per week, or suggesting he find a routine he likes to make exercise a habit. I was frustrated that he wouldn't stick to the plan or start exercising on his own.

But once I discovered that I am a Gold and he is a Saffron, the light bulb went on! Knowing my color helps me understand why I really prefer structure and routine and seem to be most consistent with exercise when I plan it in advance. But as a Saffron, he needs variety and freedom and is turned off by too much advance planning. No wonder my nagging didn't work! I was suggesting all the wrong things for him. I guess I just assumed that my approach to exercise was one that would work for anyone."

ACTIVITY

To better understand approach, turn to your specific color chapter in The 8 Colors book. Reread the four profiles in the "Meet the [fitness color]" section, and note a few of the approaches that work for each person. Which ideas and approaches might work for you?

1.

2.

3.

4.

Fitness Glossary

The Fitness Glossary matches popular activities to fitness colors. Use it as a sample guide to find activities that are likely to work for you.

And remember: It's not about the activity, it's how you go about it!

The different fitness personalities approach the same activity in particular ways that suit their personality, so pay special attention to the reasons that these particular activities are suggested.

The 8 Colors program is about the 5 Factors, not about the activity, so as you read, keep that top of mind. For instance, Blues might enjoy running or walking on familiar paths that they can measure whereas Silvers might be attracted to running or walking for the convenience and opportunity to interact with others.

Job exercisers

People who approach physical activity from the job perspective usually think of exercise as part of their overall daily or weekly plan. They feel energized by defining and completing their exercise plans. Although they may get enjoyment or satisfaction out of exercise, fun is not the motivator. Instead, motivation often comes from a sense of accomplishment by finishing their plan. Job exercisers don't necessarily avoid having others in their exercise environment, but they prefer to keep their interaction to a minimum and enjoy being with their own thoughts.

Blues, Golds, Whites, and Purples are job exercisers

Play exercisers

People who approach exercise from the play perspective usually prefer an element of fun, learning, exploration, or connection with others. They have a spontaneous nature and may feel burdened or inhibited by imposed routines, schedules, or plans. Play exercisers often gain energy by turning their attention to the outer world of the environment, and they like exercise to be disguised as something else, such as a social interaction, competition, or a way of enjoying the outdoors.

Greens, Reds, Saffrons, and Silvers are play exercisers

Job exercisers

Blues

Cardio equipment: Blues thrive in familiar and safe environments, and gravitate toward consistent routines. Treadmills, ellipticals, stationary bikes and rowing machines all allow you to easily track your progress and get down to business with minimal interruptions. You can create your own space by bringing a smartphone or book to shut out distractions.

Group fitness: Choose well-organized classes led by trainers who provide clear step-by-step instructions. Classes with predictable movements, such as spinning or strength training, will best allow you to track your progress and focus on the workout.

Rowing/boating: The solitude on the water, the rhythm and consistency of movement, and reliance on good form make rowing an excellent activity for Blues. Sailing, canoeing, and kayaking may also appeal to you — and following correct safety procedures will help you feel secure and motivated.

Running: Plan your routes ahead of time, ideally a familiar path near nature and away from busy roads. You likely prefer solo runs, and can motivate yourself with music, audiobooks, or by observing the world around you. Decide before you go whether you'll track time or distance; program your watch or app in advance.

Strength training: As a Blue, it's important for you to start slowly and master each aspect of a straightforward strength routine. You may choose to work with a qualified trainer to get comfortable with good form, after which you'll be happy to continue your routine on your own. Recording your results week by week will help keep you motivated.

Swimming: Swimming combines elements that are important to Blues — form, measuring progress, orderly lanes, and clear structure. You swim for a purpose rather than for flow or relaxation, and lap swimming provides a satisfying sense of completion.

Walking/hiking: A commonsense choice for Blues, walking is done on familiar paths and routes. You enjoy spending time in nature, alone or with a friend or family member.

Golds

Cardio equipment: Treadmills, ellipticals, stationary bikes, and rowing machines allow you to easily track progress and results. Golds seek familiarity and safety, so plan a routine and stick to it. Keep your mind engaged by watching the machine readouts. A friendly, bright, and clean fitness center is crucial.

Golf and tennis: These and other organized sports provide Golds with social time and a clear set of conventions to follow. Having a regular plan and location will give you needed structure and stability. The friendly competition may motivate you to challenge yourself and improve your fitness level.

Group fitness: Golds require a number of variables to make group fitness enjoyable. Predictable classes like spinning and strength training allow you to set and meet specific goals. Choose workouts with proven history and results (you'll likely be skeptical of the newest fads). You enjoy seeing familiar people in class, but may want to avoid overly social environments.

Running: Golds prefer familiar and safe routes with few surprises. You'll want to make a plan in advance and decide whether you'll measure distance or time. As a Gold, you are careful about injury and will stop if you experience pain. When running by yourself, keep your energy up by singing songs in your head, hashing out problems, or reciting mantras.

Strength training: It's important to find a straightforward, safe, and proven program. If you're just getting started, work with a credentialed trainer to build a routine. Track your progress over time so you can see, and share, your results.

Swimming: A favorite activity for Golds, swimming combines many important elements for you — emphasis on form, ability to feel your muscles at work, measurement, orderly lanes, and structure. You swim for purpose rather than relaxation or play.

Walking/Hiking: Golds walk with purpose, either at a fast and measurable rate for exercise, or with a friend or family member for social connection. Tracking time and distance will help motivate you; familiar routes help put you at ease.

Whites

Biking: Whites enjoy solo time on familiar bike paths. You should avoid busy traffic and the distractions/pressures of group rides. Instead opt for quiet routes and let your ride be a calm, meditative space.

Cardio machines: The repetitive motion and predictable movements of treadmills, ellipticals, and stationary bikes allow your mind to wander and explore. Research and create a plan ahead of time, and opt for orderly and uncrowded fitness centers.

Running: Running is a natural fit for you, especially if you follow planned, familiar routes that inflict minimal interruptions. Quiet, solitary runs in natural settings are best.

Swimming: The calm, repetitive motion and feel of the water help your mind relax, enabling you to savor ideas and thoughts that rise from your unconscious.

Strength training: Do your research and create a plan that will challenge you. You may appreciate circuit classes that break things down into component parts; choose familiar environments and trusted instructors so you feel comfortable. Once you have a plan, stick to it and work in a quiet environment that will allow you to get into a flow.

Tai Chi: This ancient moving meditation fits well with your desire for peacefulness and intention. Look for small classes in calm and/or outdoor settings. Search for an instructor you are comfortable with and respect.

Walking/hiking: Familiar and tranquil routes will hold the most appeal for you. Embrace the solitude of nature on solo hikes, allowing yourself to take a break from the everyday world and let your mind wander free.

Yoga: The mind-body connection will appeal to you, especially the deep learning and practice of yoga. Classes allow for some companionship without too much socializing, or you can practice in the peaceful solitude of your home.

Purples

Biking: Purples typically ride on a few planned routes and enjoy biking alone. Avoid distractions, such as busy traffic or keeping pace with others. The quiet rotation of the bike wheels will help carry you to a calm and meditative space.

Cardio equipment: Treadmills, ellipticals, and stationary bikes allow you to select a program and stick to it. You can follow your plan with ease, even in unfamiliar fitness centers. Having people around can give you a boost of energy, and watching TV or listening to music helps pass the time.

Pilates: Purples are drawn to the organization and targeted results you get from a Pilates workout. Pilates is also great for posture, which is likely important to you.

Running: As a Purple, you are most comfortable following planned, familiar routes and running by yourself or with a quiet companion. The calming, repetitive motion allows your active mind to drift miles away. For variety, you might enjoy an occasional group run.

Strength training: Purples methodically organize weight routines to hit each muscle group. You can likely devise a plan for yourself (or with the help of a competent trainer). Once you're familiar with the routine, TV or music can help pass the time. For variety and a challenge, you could try a carefully paced group class.

Swimming: The calm, repetitive motion and the feel of the water help your mind relax. The order and structure of lap swimming put you at ease. Keep track of progress with a clock or by counting laps so you know when you've completed your workout.

Walking/hiking: As a Purple, walking and hiking can take many different forms. Depending on your mood and goals, your walks can be leisurely or aerobic, social or introspective.

Yoga: Yoga provides solitude within a group setting, and a regular class can help satisfy your desire for routine (plus you can check off the flexibility box). Because you already have insight into your internal world, the spiritual aspects of yoga may or may not appeal.

Play exercisers

Greens

Activities of daily life: Find every opportunity you can to be active during day-to-day life. Park farther from your destination, walk instead of drive, or take the stairs. Outdoor chores are especially motivating for you — yard work, gardening, putting up fences, or chopping wood.

Biking: Solo, outdoor rides (with minimal planning) are your best opportunity to savor the experience, whether road or mountain biking. If you're on the practical side, you might bike to work instead of driving.

Running: You appreciate the convenience and solitude of solo runs in the outdoors. Observing every detail of the world around you will keep you engaged. Leave music and other distractions at home, which will only make you feel over stimulated.

Strength training: Greens will often set up creative drills and obstacles courses, like a backyard ropes course. You'll have the most fun with creative outdoor strength training.

Swimming: Water in natural settings has a strong draw. Rivers, oceans, lakes, and ponds allow you to explore entire underwater worlds. You may train for a specific event with lap swimming.

Walking/hiking: A natural fit for the nature-loving Greens, walking or hiking is an easy and convenient opportunity for you to get outdoors. Use your outstanding observational skills to take in the subtle changes in your environment over time.

Windsurfing/sailboarding: These water activities bring you as close to nature as you can get, merging with the water and the wind. The challenge and thrill combines all the elements that appeal to you: sensory experience, alone time, and the natural world.

Reds

Biking: Mountain or road biking is an effective way for you to explore the outdoors, get your heart rate up, and challenge yourself. Find people to ride with who are at your level and will keep you from getting bored during a ride.

Cardio machines: If you must workout indoors, seek out a machine with a view of the outdoors. You can make the experience more fun by competing against a friend or by training for an adventurous fitness challenge.

Group fitness: Choose classes that are high energy, fun, and sociable. Look for fitness centers with a variety of classes where you can drop in as your schedule and whims allow. Find upbeat instructors with great taste in music.

Running: Get outdoors and enjoy spontaneous (or causally planned) runs with your friends. You can keep energy up by setting mini goals for yourself and competing against yourself or others. Make sure to have your running gear close at hand for when the opportunity presents itself.

Strength training: Your strength routine should feel fun and geared toward measurable results. Find workout buddies at a similar level, and add motivation by working with an upbeat trainer who will give you plenty of feedback in the moment.

Team sports: Fast-paced, fun, and competitive sports like basketball, racquetball, and tennis will keep you interested. Choose games where you can funnel your high energy, quick reflexes, and intensity, while still having fun. Casually planned or spur-of-the-moment pickup games will work better for you than highly structured sports leagues.

Walking/hiking: Requiring minimal planning, this is a great way to invest in your physical activity while connecting with your friends and family. Get "lost" in nature and observe the world around you. Play games along the way to infuse the experience with a sense of fun and competition.

Saffrons

Biking: You appreciate the convenience of starting a ride from your front door (make sure your bike is tuned up and ready to go). Biking can be peaceful and challenging, providing transportation or an opportunity to explore the outdoors. Riding with others can be fun as long as there's minimal coordination.

Cardio equipment: You're unlikely to regularly use cardio machines at a fitness center — unless it's part of a specific training program. The novelty of "exergaming" systems can add a level of fun and competition to otherwise boring machines.

Dancing: Saffrons have an innate love of flow and music, which makes dance a natural fit. Try many types of dance — salsa, folk, flamenco, swing, and ballroom. Drop-in classes with minimal structure will feel the most fun.

Group fitness: Saffrons enjoy fun classes that encourage self expression. Look for a fitness center with flexible offerings that allow you to attend class when time opens up (keep a gym bag ready). Good music and a fun instructor are essential.

Martial arts: This diverse group of traditions involve flow, concentration, and discipline — all of which appeal to Saffrons. Look for small group classes and an instructor you connect with. You may also be inspired by exploring the philosophy behind the tradition you choose.

Running: Running can be done anywhere and requires little advanced planning, so keep your sneakers close at hand. Avoid boredom by finding a good partner: someone at your level with a flexible schedule (who's not too chatty). When alone, music will keep your energy up. Training for an event can also motivate you.

Walking/hiking: Walking or hiking allows you to enjoy the freedom of the outdoors with minimal coordination. It can be done virtually anywhere and requires only a good pair of shoes. You prefer walking alone or with a small group.

Yoga: Saffrons gravitate toward yoga for the mind-body connection. This practice offers spiritual depth, stresses balance and peacefulness, and provides an ongoing challenge. An outstanding teacher is a must.

Silvers

Biking: The convenience of starting a ride from your front door makes biking a natural choice. Scheduled group rides can also provide the consistency you need to fit biking into your hectic life, while adding a social element that helps distract you from the monotony of exercise.

Cardio equipment: You prefer to get your cardio workouts outdoors, but will use a machine as a backup. Meeting friends at the gym and planning something fun for after the workout can help motivate you. Arrive at the gym dressed and ready to go to avoid unnecessary obstacles like talking to people.

Dancing: With your flair for drama, and love of music and self expression, you may enjoy many types of dance. Salsa, folk, flamenco, swing, and ballroom can be great fitness options.

Group fitness: Look for fun and social classes. Flexibility is important for you, so find a fitness center that has a variety of classes where you can drop in as your schedule allows. A positive instructor and upbeat playlist will help distract you.

Running: Running requires minimal process and can be done anywhere. This activity provides the biggest bang for your buck — an important consideration with your busy life. Running with others is a great way for you to socialize, maintain accountability, and keep up your momentum.

Strength training: Straightforward programs can be boring for you, so look for interesting and sociable environments. This is most likely accomplished by working with a trainer, or by disguising exercise through activities such as yoga and Pilates.

Walking/hiking: One of the most convenient activities, it can be done virtually anywhere and requires only a good pair of shoes. Walking also gives you opportunities to explore your environment. Keep coordination for group outings simple.

Yoga and Tai Chi: Silvers gravitate toward yoga and tai chi for the mind-body connection. These practices provide intellectual and spiritual interest while stressing balance and peacefulness. Taking a regular group class will help keep you accountable and committed.

Choose effective thoughts

ACTIVITY

As you have been discovering in this program, each color has unique preferences for a physically active lifestyle. One of the easiest ways to become disconnected from these preferences is through habitual negative thinking or ineffective thoughts.

As you read through the list, place a mark by any ineffective phrases that you've thought in the past. Then beside each ineffective phrase, write a more effective statement you could use that would help you shift into an effective thinking cycle. At the bottom of this activity, add any other ineffective thoughts that might keep you stuck and replace them with more effective ones.

INEFFECTIVE	EFFECTIVE
I know I should exercise, but I hate it, so I just can't seem to make myself do it.	**Example statement:** Being physically active doesn't mean doing exercise just for the sake of exercise. If I think of it like that, I'll never do it! Instead, I can focus on ways to be active in nature because I love the outdoors. **Your effective statement:**
I don't know if exercise is really worth the effort.	**Example statement:** Although the list of medical benefits of exercise doesn't inspire me, I know exercise always helps free me up from internal stress – and that's worth the effort! **Your effective statement:**
I don't have time.	**Example statement:** Since my time is tight, I can choose activities that start at my front door and not waste time driving to and from a gym. Plus, if I pair it with socializing with someone I enjoy, I'll feel like my time is well spent. **Your effective statement:**

I'm too embarrassed to be seen exercising.

Example statement: For now, I can focus on exercising in my house with fitness videos because I really enjoy exercising by myself anyway. Over time, I'll feel more comfortable exercising in front of other people if I choose to do that.

Your effective statement:

I can't do what they recommend, so why bother?

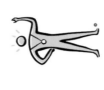

Example statement: I don't like to follow exercise guidelines. But I love activities that are social and competitive. To get myself back in the game, I'll check with the local recreation center about their softball league schedules.

Your effective statement:

I was doing pretty well until I got sick (or busy, or company visited, or I went on vacation, or ...)

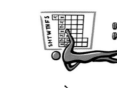

Example statement: I can think of this like a work project that got interrupted. To get back on track, I need to clarify my goals again, develop a plan, and get it on the calendar.

Your effective statement:

I started exercising, but I quit because I wasn't seeing the weight loss I expected.

Example statement: I know if I stick with it, the weight will come off eventually. Until then, I can focus on other things that are really important to me, like being a good role model for my children and improving my walking pace.

Your effective statement:

I used to be so athletic. Now I'm just out of shape and lazy.

Example statement: I'm not trying to compete in sports. I just want to be independent and take care of myself as long as possible. Being active will help me do that.

Your effective statement:

UNDERSTANDING FOCUS AND MENTAL ENGAGEMENT

The third of the five factors of fitness personality is focus: what engages your mind while exercising.

FACTOR 3 Focus

Focus is the "what?" of your fitness program.

Creating a program that helps you remain engaged will make staying with it much easier. To understand your focus, ask yourself:

- What do I like to pay attention to?
- What helps me get the mental stimulation necessary to stick with my workout program?
- What decreases my energy or momentum?

For example:

- Greens enjoy connecting with what's in front of them, savoring the details and small variations in nature.
- Whites are energized by activities that allow for internal reflection and opportunities to zone out.

In this section, you'll identify your own preferred focus during physical activity. We'll also explore a highly effective method for taking your first steps toward your fitness goals: the 4-Day Win.

Each of the eight fitness colors has its own preferred focus for each of the eight colors. In addition to reading the list for your own color, read the lists for the colors that are next to yours on the color wheel. As you read the three lists, circle any phrases that describe you.

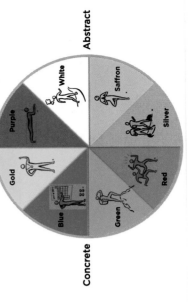

Color-Specific Focus: What Engages Your Mind?

Blue

- Focusing on correct form and proper technique
- Concentrating on chanting, mantras, or songs
- Monitoring and measuring shorter- and longer-term exercise goals
- Reading or listening to audio recordings

Gold

- Focusing on correct form and proper technique
- Concentrating on chanting, mantras, or songs
- Monitoring and measuring shorter- and longer-term exercise goals
- Listening to music or watching TV

White

- Attending to internal thoughts and letting things "pop up"
- Engaging in repetitive motion to zone out
- Enjoying familiar surroundings and predictable activities
- Reading or listening to audio recordings when engaged in routine cardio activities

Purple

- Attending to internal thoughts and letting things "pop up"
- Using repetitive motion as an opportunity to zone out
- Focusing on time, distance, or completing planned workout
- Reading, listening to audio recordings, or watching TV during cardio workouts

Green

- Using outstanding direction and observation skills
- Taking in the physical surroundings, including smells and sounds
- Responding to activities and actions
- Noticing details in nature

Red

- Taking in the physical surroundings, including smells and sounds
- Responding to activities and actions
- Having a goal to provide focus and relieve boredom
- Listening to energetic music or watching action TV during cardio workouts at the gym

Saffron

- Listening to music while active
- Having a challenge or a goal to focus on
- Directing attention on an activity while getting exercise along the way
- Having fun because exercise is boring by itself

Silver

- Learning something new and interesting
- Having a challenge or a goal to focus on
- Directing attention on an activity while getting exercise along the way
- Focusing on the mind-body connection

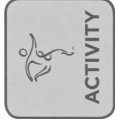

ACTIVITY

Put your preferences into practice

Creating positive experiences during exercise is key to getting and keeping the motivation you need to stick to your physical activity plan. As you work toward a steady physical activity program, it's important to understand and connect with your preferences. Friends, family members, and others may try to help you create your program, but their help may not always match your true fitness color. Be sure to stay focused on the strategies that support your true color.

The following activity will help you discover how to use your personal focus effectively. In the left column, choose the fitness color focus from the previous page that best describes you. Next to the focus, describe how you'll put it into action.

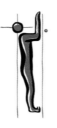

FOCUS

Example from a Purple:

1. Engage in repetitive motion to zone out

HOW YOU'LL USE IT

1. Find out the hours at the YMCA pool. Create a plan to swim there before work several days per week, and use swim time for reflection and to get my creative juices going.
2. Find a familiar route to walk that will allow me to get my workout in without paying attention to where I'm going.

THE 4-DAY WIN

Prochaska stresses the need to set very small, attainable goals as you work to make a change. These goals help build your confidence and create slow but steady momentum.

Martha Beck, life coach and best-selling author, has found in her coaching work that many clients balk at a week-long program of change but are willing to try something new for four days. With such a short span of time to work with, large goals have to be broken down into tiny, manageable ones. At the end of the four days, even though they are told that they can stop, most of her clients continue, seeing positive changes and realizing that they have already overcome their initial resistance. The 4-Day Win has proven to be an effective tool whether you're trying to start an exercise program, lose weight, stop smoking, or make other changes.

Break down your goal

You might not be ready at this point in the program to imagine meeting the CDC guidelines. But you can picture yourself making small changes for just four days, and they will move you toward success. Small changes can have a positive effect on your motivation, leading you to make more changes.

According to Beck, the "win" is the sense of accomplishment that motivates you to keep working on your goal for another four days.

Beck advises paring down goals again and again until they are small enough to accomplish in four days. Instead of overwhelming yourself by saying, "I will become a more physically active person," you say instead, "I will walk for 30 minutes each day." If that still feels unrealistic, pare it down until, as Beck says, your goal is "ridiculously easy to attain." For example, walking to the receptionist instead of using the intercom or walking around the kitchen while boiling water.

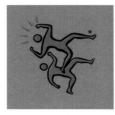

JIM, A RED, NATURALLY FOCUSES ON THE EXTERNAL WORLD AND IS ALWAYS IN THE MOMENT. HE DESCRIBES THE DIFFERENCE BETWEEN HIMSELF AND THOSE WHO ENJOY A QUIETER, MORE INTERNAL FOCUS:

"For me, it's perfect that I live near a recreation center with outdoor basketball courts because I can go down there any night of the week and find at least a few guys to shoot hoops with. I mostly enjoy exercise when it's fast paced and I'm in the action. When I see people in the gym pedaling a stationary bike and reading, I think, 'How can they stand to do that?' That type of exercise just isn't for me."

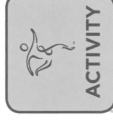

ACTIVITY

Create your own 4-day Win

1. **Choose a four-day goal that's a small step toward your overall goal.**
If your overall goal, for example, is to meet the CDC guidelines and do 150 minutes of moderate aerobic activity each week, start with a 20 minute walk for four days.

2. **Break it down.** Think you can't — or won't — be able to accomplish that goal? Make it smaller. Keep your current level of fitness in mind, and pick a goal that feels easy to attain. How about a 10 minute brisk walk each day?

3. **Repeat the process.** Once you complete your first 4-Day Win, slightly increase your next goal and keep the momentum going! Continue to reward yourself as you take small steps toward your overall goal.

Are you ready for change?

We don't all start the process of change at the same stage, and we don't move through the stages at the same pace. Each of the five stages brings unique challenges and rewards, and trying to jump ahead or move through them too quickly can hurt your chances of long-term success. Remember, change is all about decisional balance, increasing the pros and reducing the cons.

Note:

There are no right or wrong stages — each is important and part of the process!

Know your stage

Review the following five statements and select the one that best describes you at this moment. Then circle the name of the stage to the right of the statement.

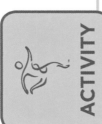

ACTIVITY

I'm not considering becoming more physically active right now, or I'm considering it but don't think I'm likely to make the change now.

1. NOT CONSIDERING

I'm considering becoming more physically active in the next six months.

2. CONSIDERING

I'm preparing to become more physically active within the next 30 days.

3. PREPARING

I'm presently engaging in physical activity.

4. ENGAGING

I've made physical activity a habit and have been maintaining this habit for six months.

5. MAINTAINING

Use this page to reflect on what you've learned, both about The 8 Colors program and about yourself.

Consider the following questions as a guide:

Which of the color-specific approaches and focuses inspire you? Describe.

What self-defeating thoughts might get in the way of your progress?

What have you learned this week that might explain why you haven't successfully maintained an exercise program in the past?

What fitness activities are you excited about?

Are you starting a 4-Day Win? How will you break it down to truly make it a win?

Other....

Use this white space for your notes!

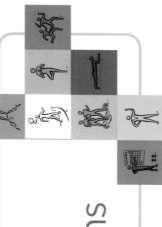

CHAPTER 4

environment and interpersonal connections

Welcome to week four! Now that you've discovered your color-coded motivation, approach, and focus, and you've completed your first 4-Day Win, the next step is to explore the fourth and fifth factors of your fitness personality: environment and interpersonal connections. You'll see how important choosing the right environment is to long-term success, and you'll identify the level or type of involvement with others you prefer while exercising. In addition, you will develop personalized strategies for your own barriers.

FACTOR 4

Environment

Environment is the "where?" of physical activity.

Many environments facilitate activity, and choosing the right one(s) for your color is the key to maintaining your energy. Do you mostly enjoy the outdoors? Would you rather go to a fitness center or work out at home? Do you prefer a combination of the two?

For example:

- Purples enjoy the many offerings of a well-organized fitness center.
- Greens recharge their batteries outside.

On the next page, you'll find highlights of the preferred environments for each of the eight fitness colors. In addition to reading the list for your own color, read the lists for the colors that are next to yours on the color wheel. As you read the three lists, circle any phrases that describe you.

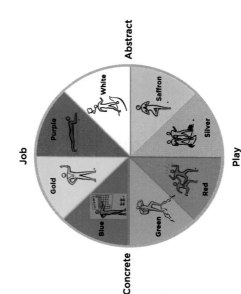

Color-Specific Environment: Where do you most enjoy being physically active?

Blue

- Outdoor environments that are safe and predictable
- Familiar environments — same time, same place
- Fitness centers where I can get in and out quickly
- Fitness centers where I can create my own space by using headphones or reading

Gold

- Outdoor environments that are safe and predictable
- Familiar environments — same time, same place
- Fitness centers that are open and well lit
- Gyms with an organized and friendly atmosphere

Purple

- Outdoor environments with familiar paths and routes
- New environments for variety and convenience
- Fitness centers with many choices of activities and amenities
- Fitness centers with an organized and friendly atmosphere

White

- Peaceful and calm environments
- Small, quiet, and uncrowded fitness centers
- Fitness centers that I have checked out prior to beginning my workout
- Outdoor environments with familiar paths and routes

Green

- Outdoors in nature
- Fitness center if in preparation for an important outdoor event
- Anywhere I can have fun using my outstanding navigational skills
- The highest point for the best scenery and views

Red

- Outdoors in nature
- Anywhere high energy and action packed
- Well-lit gyms offering cardio equipment with a view
- At home, with fitness equipment in sight

Saffron

- Outdoors in natural surroundings and fresh air
- Easily accessible environment with few barriers to getting started
- Outdoors when doing cardio activities
- Fitness centers with a casual atmosphere and dress code

Silver

- Outdoors in natural surroundings and fresh air
- Easily accessible environment with few barriers to getting started
- Anywhere that offers many choices of activities/times
- New environments where I can explore and get exercise along the way

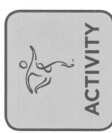

Put your preferences into practice

No matter what type of environment you like to exercise in, you can use your preferences to create your best strategies and experiences. Friends, family members, and others may try to help you create your program, but their help may not always match your true fitness color. Be sure to stay focused on the strategies that support your true color.

The following activity will help you discover how to use your environment preferences effectively. In the left column, choose the environment from the previous page that best describes you. Next to the environment, describe how you'll incorporate it into your life.

PREFERENCE

Example from a Blue:

1. Fitness Centers where I can get in and out quickly

HOW YOU'LL USE IT

1. Get recommendations about fitness centers from a coworker

2. Visit fitness centers that are convenient to walk to or have good parking

3. Try before you buy. Help find the right fitness center by taking advantage of one week free pass offered by most fitness centers

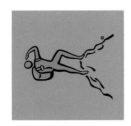

JEFF, A GREEN, MAKES HIS ENVIRONMENTAL PREFERENCES CLEAR:

"I love being in nature as much as possible. There's so much to see and experience. When going for a walk outdoors, I usually take my binoculars and identify plants, birds, and animals along the way. I notice the rocks, where trees have fallen, and how wide the trail is compared to other trails. I'm frequently bored inside, but never bored outside."

UNDERSTANDING INTERPERSONAL CONNECTIONS

The fifth factor of fitness personality is interpersonal connections: who you exercise with, your level of or type of involvement with others while exercising.

FACTOR 5 Interpersonal Connections

Interpersonal connections is the "who?" of your fitness program.

For some fitness colors, working out with others provides fun, momentum, and accountability. For others, working out alone is desirable and energizing.

For example:

- Internally motivated Blues prefer routine exercise with minimal interaction with others.
- Training with others stimulates Reds, and their energy diminishes when they are alone.

Fitness research shows that your chances of exercising regularly increase when you are in a culture that supports an active lifestyle. Having friends, families, and colleagues who are physically active — no matter their fitness preferences — makes it more likely that you will stick with your program.

NOTE: Although all fitness colors can successfully and occasionally work out with a partner or in a group, some colors prefer little to no interaction with others, and may be put off by the thought of an "exercise buddy."

To make working out with others successful for all personalities, you need a shared understanding about what each person needs and wants from the other. Some colors are natural partners and can exercise together seamlessly. Some colors who are not natural workout buddies will do well together in an activity or sport that is out of the ordinary for both.

Put your preferences into practice

You can use your preferences to create your best strategies and experiences, whether you like to interact with people during exercise or not. Friends, family members, and others may try to help you with suggestions about how you should include others, but their help may not match your true fitness color. Be sure to stay focused on the strategies that support your true color.

The Buddy System – Make it work for you

Because we naturally approach exercise more from either a job or play viewpoint, here are some helpful tips for both types of exercisers:

Job Exercisers

- Remember, it's OK to let others know you prefer to keep exercise as your "alone time."
- Exercising with others may be challenging for you, especially if you have time constraints.
- If you exercise with others, choose activities that require less interaction.
- If you train for an event with others or join a team, also allow time for independent exercise.

Play Exercisers

- Look for exercise buddies you are likely to have fun with in general.
- Use exercise as a time to be with friends and family.
- Incorporate exercise into productive activities, such as walking meetings with colleagues.
- Keep your workout gear handy so you are ready for impromptu opportunities.

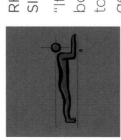

RHONDA, A PURPLE, DESCRIBES THE SUBTLE DIFFERENCE BETWEEN HER SISTER SANDY, A SILVER, AND HERSELF:

"It works for Sandy and me to go to the gym together because we're both clear on our differences and don't expect to actually be exercising together. She needs the accountability of a set time and date with me to get herself there, and I like the variety of going with someone else rather than exercising on my own all the time. But once we actually get to the gym, we do very different things. She likes to lift weights and chat with people in the main part of the workout room while I'm more likely to zone out by myself on a cardio machine. We meet up when we're both done and head home together."

Color-Specific Interpersonal Connections: Who do you exercise with?

Below, you'll find a review of the preferred interpersonal connections for each of the eight fitness colors. In addition to reading the list for your own color, read the lists for the colors that are next to yours on the color wheel. As you read the three lists, circle any phrases that describe you.

It's important to note that your preferences for interpersonal connections are heavily influenced by whether you're a job or play exerciser. For guidance on whether you should consider working out with an exercise buddy, refer to page 14 in Chapter 1.

Purple

- Working out alone is energizing
- Prefer to keep exercising and socializing separate
- Enjoy having other people in the environment, but not interacting directly
- Exercise near or alongside others for variety

Silver

- Coordinated exercise with others creates accountability
- Including others in physical activity makes it fun and helps pass the time
- Can think and plan when exercising alone

White

- Working out alone is energizing
- Enjoy peaceful, quiet setting
- Find unwanted chit-chat irritating
- Might work out with a few others as long as goals can be achieved according to plan

Saffron

- Attracted to independent activities alongside other people
- Enjoy sports with others that are easily coordinated and fun
- Keeps momentum high by light conversation with others
- Can think and plan when exercising alone

Gold

- Enjoy having people in the environment, but not interacting directly
- Take pleasure in sharing accomplishments with others
- Attracted to socializing around organized sporting activities
- Might work out with others as long as goals can be achieved according to plan

Red

- Playing sports with others is a way of life
- Competing inspires better performance and is fun
- Interacting with others keeps the momentum high and beats the boredom

Blue

- Working out alone is energizing
- Prefer keeping exercise and socializing separate
- Focus on meeting their goals and avoid the distractions of others
- Might work out with a few others if goals can be achieved according to plan

Green

- Enjoy being alone in nature
- Exercising solo enables flexibility
- Prefer training for a goal alone
- Competing with others inspires better performance and is fun

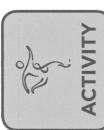

ACTIVITY

Put your preferences into practice

As you are learning, there are many ways to approach interpersonal connections when it comes to fitness. Now that you have an introduction to the different preferences of the eight fitness colors, use this information to explore what sort of social interaction might work for you.

The following activity will help you discover how to use your preferred interpersonal connections effectively. In the left column, choose interpersonal connections from the previous page that best describe you. Next to the interpersonal connections, describe how you'll put them into action.

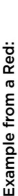

INTERPERSONAL CONNECTIONS

Example from a Red:

HOW YOU'LL USE IT

1. Competing with others inspires better performance and is fun.

1. Investigate the basketball league in the area
2. Train for a 5k run with friends or family

THE BUDDY SYSTEM

Blues

Gold
- Golds are equally comfortable with advanced planning
- Find Blues at your level
- Get the job done and socialize afterwards
- Golds can be chatty, which may be distracting for you

Blue
- Plan ahead and rely on a regular routine
- Share tips on good form
- Ideal for quiet companionship

Green
- You make the plans and tell your Green friend to just show up
- Spend time outdoors
- Greens may happily help with yard chores, moving, and daily life activities

Red
- Reds will draw you out of your comfort zone
- They prefer spontaneity; last minute invites are OK
- Try a team sport together

Purple
- Purples will introduce you to new things or try a fitness class with you
- An occasional, casual workout buddy
- Agree on time or distance ahead of time

White
- Whites will be quiet, reliable fitness buddies
- An occasional add-on for both of you
- Peacefully do your own thing in the same space

Saffron
- Saffrons bring a sense of play
- Treat as a supplement to your normal workouts
- Nice change of pace if you let go of your agenda

Silver
- Will try new activities with you
- You'll be keeping measurements for both of you
- Silvers will welcome you doing the planning

Golds

Purple
- Purple friends can help you cross-train
- You're both chatty but serious about your workouts
- Find Purples at your level
- Separate at the gym and socialize afterward

White
- Choose activities that require little interaction
- Whites may be more reserved conversationalists
- Meet your White friends where they are comfortable

Saffron
- Team sports are a fun choice for this pair
- Choose activities that take pressure off the social interaction
- You'll do most of the talking

Silver
- Silvers offer camaraderie, conversation and enthusiasm
- Silvers will encourage you to try new things
- Don't expect them to adhere to your routine
- Good training buddies for an event (vs. regular workouts)

Gold
- Amiable, good-spirited workout buddies
- You're both happy to cheer each other on
- Set goals and share your accomplishments

Blue
- Try training for a specific event together
- Blues might want less interaction
- Consistent, steady training partner

Green
- Nature activities are a sure bet
- Encourage Green friends to share observations
- Let go of your plans and follow them into the wilderness

Red
- Reds may seem overly competitive or risky
- They can push you to reach new goals
- You'll do the planning
- They're up for last-minute invites

Purples

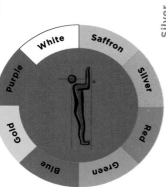

Gold
- Bring goals for the workout that you can share
- Work out separately and socialize afterward
- You're both comfortable sticking to plans

Blue
- You can learn from Blue's attention to form
- They can help you focus
- Blues are enjoyable companions who won't distract from the workout

Green
- Relax and let Green guide you on a nature hike or climb
- If there's an outdoor activity you've been reluctant to try, go with your Green friend

Red
- Reds can provide exciting new adventures
- They'll help you be in the moment
- Watch for Red's competitive drive, which may make you uncomfortable

Purple
- Choose fitness classes in which you can each do your own thing
- Train for same event, but train by yourself
- Meeting up after a workout is nice

White
- You'll be energized by working out in proximity
- Choose known fitness centers or routes
- It's OK to meet there and do your own thing

Saffron
- Don't treat your shared activity as a serious workout
- Saffrons are looking for fun
- Great source for workout music

Silver
- Silvers are always game to try something new
- This is your buddy for trying something really out of the ordinary (kayaking trip, mountain climbing, etc.)

Whites

Gold
- Golds can help you snap out of research mode
- Gold's chattiness can be irritating for you
- Establish goals in advance and separate when you want to get the job done.

Blue
- Blues' quiet focus works well with your desire for peacefulness
- Socializing will happen outside of the workout
- Blues won't demand your attention

Green
- Greens can help you be present to the world around you
- Make plans with a start and end time
- You're both quiet and appreciate peacefulness

Red
- Invite Reds to play with you in a sport you enjoy
- When communicating plans, keep it brief and direct
- Don't be put-off by Reds' tendency to make everything into a competition

Purple
- Can introduce you to new experiences
- You need more transition time, so arrive separately
- Invite your Purple friend to a class you already attend

White
- Honor your type, and let each other do your own thing
- Share ideas after the workout
- You're both independent and enjoy solitude, you're unlikely to look for a fitness buddy

Saffron
- Choose a space that's familiar to both of you
- You both likely prefer the outdoors
- This pairing will be more friendship than fitness

Silver
- Be prepared for Silver's high social energy
- You might enjoy listening to their ideas during a workout
- Invite them for a walking meeting

Gold

- Invite Golds to join you for outdoor activities
- They'll love to hear your observations
- Be prepared for them to be chatty

Blue

- Blue friends will want to plan in advance
- Offer to help your Blue pals with chores, moving, or yard work
- You're both quiet

Green

- Matching minimalist approach
- Fellow Greens will be happy to hike in silence
- Compare gear tips and discuss the latest research

Red

- Reds will challenge you and bring out your competitive side
- You'll have fun together, on occasion
- Reds will be game for a spontaneous outing

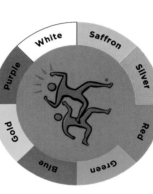

Purple

- Share the outdoors with your Purple friends
- Swap ideas and observations
- Purples may want to be more chatty

White

- You can be quiet together
- Meet for simple, calm outdoor activities
- Your natural GPS will put your White friends at ease

Saffron

- Skip the gym and share outdoor experiences
- Your saffron friends will love hearing your observations about the world
- Well matched with pace, energy, and spontaneity

Silver

- Be ready — Silvers will bring a high level of energy
- They'll want to learn from you and hear your observations
- Shorter engagements are better

Gold

- Golds are friendly, outgoing, and make great sports buddies
- They can help you moderate your risk taking
- They'll be happy to swap mutual accomplishments

Blue

- Make plans to play a team sport together
- Blue's focus on safety and moderation will help keep you from going overboard
- Blues will keep track of time and distance

Green

- Greens will have unusual training tips to share
- They'll turn down regular invites but enjoy getting together occasionally
- Greens are up for a text with a last-minute plan

Red

- You both love friendly competition
- You'll both have your gear ready for an adventure at a moment's notice
- Don't push each other too far

Purple

- Purples will be game to join you on fun outings (at least once)
- They'll keep you engaged
- May not share your drive for competition

White

- Whites will help moderate your impulse to go all out
- Less social than you, but will actually find you funny
- Join your White friend in their preferred space

Saffron

- Saffrons share your sense of fun and adventure
- Saffrons might disappear if you become too competitive
- Will join you in an offbeat activity

Silver

- Silvers are great workout buddies
- Choose activities that are interactive and social
- Challenge them to higher levels with your competitive spirit

Saffrons

Gold
- Golds are great cheerleaders and can help distract you
- You take a more casual approach than Gold friends
- They'll share form tips if asked
- They may be overly eager to offer advice

Blue
- Blues enjoy advanced planning; not spontaneous
- They'll share tips if asked
- You need to feel quite simpatico with this person for it to work

Green
- Well matched in terms of energy, spontaneity, and your love of the outdoors
- Greens will share their observations and keep you engaged

Red
- Reds can be fun and inspiring training partners
- They're ready to go whenever you are
- Reds may be too competitive for your tastes

Purple
- Purples prefer to exercise alone
- You could try an out-of-the-routine experience
- May turn down your workout invite and join you afterward for socializing

White
- You share an intellectual bond
- Activities will be more about friendship than fitness
- Find peaceful environments and outdoor activities

Saffron
- You share the desire to have fun and be challenged
- Minimal coordination and convenience are musts
- Choose activities that will disguise exercise

Silver
- Silvers provide easy conversation and distraction
- They can broaden your horizons
- Keep equipment handy so you're ready for last-minute invites

Silvers

Gold
- Energy levels well matched
- Will provide accountability for you to show up
- They can help break down a workout into accomplishable pieces

Blue
- Blues can offer accountability
- You'll probably have to initiate,
- Blues not looking for workout buddies
- Blues will be open to walking meetings

Green
- Greens will share their observations and keep you engaged
- Be careful not to overtake the conversation
- Greens will keep you safe
- Up for last-minute plans

Red
- Reds will push you to higher levels
- They'll provide challenges and excitement
- Choose activities that are interactive and social

Purple
- You may enjoy taking yoga or another class together
- Purples mostly workout solo
- They'll try something new with you

White
- White can make a good sport buddy
- You'll be doing most of the talking
- They want familiar — join Whites where they are

Saffron
- Can provide great conversation for each other
- OK with last minute planning or cancellation
- Saffrons are game for new adventures
- Prefer the outdoors

Silver
- You can feed into each other's mutual desire for momentum
- Silvers can effectively distract each other from exercise
- May not be the best serious training partner
- You'll have fun talking with each other

NOTES

Use this page to reflect on what you've learned, both about The 8 Colors program and about yourself.

Consider the following questions as a guide:

Which of the color-specific environments supports your physical activity? Why?

How do you prefer to be involved with others (or not) while exercising? How might this add to your enjoyment?

What have you learned this week that might explain why you haven't successfully maintained an exercise program in the past?

Other....

Use this white space for your notes!

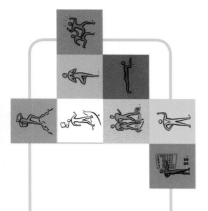

CHAPTER 5   putting it all together

Don't forget to use the white space!

Welcome to week five! Over the last four weeks, you've moved closer to a program of regular physical activity. You know **why** you are motivated, **how** you best approach exercise, **what** engages your mind, **where** you like to exercise, and with **whom**. You also have many of the tools you need to get started. The next step is to develop a specific plan to help you achieve long-term success.

In this chapter, we'll also look at color-specific barriers, the barriers that can zap your commitment.

Moving Forward

Your goal four weeks ago was to create an exercise program that you could stick with. During those weeks, you've learned how to do that, beginning with identifying your fitness personality and then discovering the unique preferences of your personality. You've also assessed where you are in the Stages of Change model and explored ways to move through those stages.

Are you ready for change?

Let's reassess where you stand, keeping in mind that you might still be at the same stage, but noting any shifts in thinking or behaviors that indicate progress. Remember that trying to jump ahead or move through the stages too quickly can hurt your chances of long-term success.

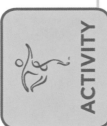

ACTIVITY

Know your stage

Review the following five statements and select the one that best describes you at this moment. Then circle the name of the stage to the right of the statement.

Note:
There are no right or wrong stages — each is important and part of the process!

I'm not considering becoming more physically active right now, or I'm considering it but don't think I'm likely to make the change now.

1. NOT CONSIDERING

I'm considering becoming more physically active in the next six months.

2. CONSIDERING

I'm preparing to become more physically active within the next 30 days.

3. PREPARING

I'm presently engaging in physical activity.

4. ENGAGING

I've made physical activity a habit and have been maintaining this habit for six months.

5. MAINTAINING

Common Barriers

This section will help you understand common color-specific barriers and identify how these barriers may appear in your life. You'll be more likely to stay with your program if you can anticipate, recognize, and prepare for them in advance.

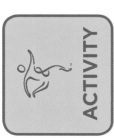

ACTIVITY

What are your barriers?

Below you'll find a list of the most common barriers for each of the eight fitness colors. In addition to reading the list for your own color, read the lists for the colors that are next to yours on the color wheel. As you read the three lists, check any barriers you think you might face along your journey to a more active lifestyle.

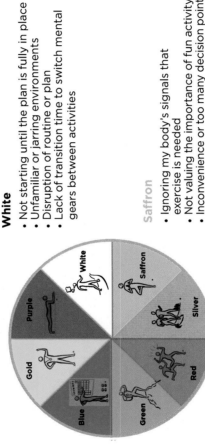

Gold
- Safety concerns
- Lacking clear goals for physical activity
- Not scheduling activity in advance
- Disruption of routine or plan

Blue
- Not scheduling activity in advance
- Other responsibilities that could take priority
- Over-stimulating or disorganized environments
- Disruption of routine or plan

Green
- Boredom of routine exercise
- Not getting outside into nature
- Missing chances to include activity in my daily living
- Difficulty finding time alone to exercise

Red
- Boredom of routine exercise
- Lack of people to connect with during exercise
- Not having a goal
- Not getting outdoors

Purple
- Trying to exercise without a plan
- Distracting or jarring environments
- Interruptions to my exercise plan
- Not making exercise a part of my lifestyle

White
- Not starting until the plan is fully in place
- Unfamiliar or jarring environments
- Disruption of routine or plan
- Lack of transition time to switch mental gears between activities

Saffron
- Ignoring my body's signals that exercise is needed
- Not valuing the importance of fun activity
- Inconvenience or too many decision points
- Getting sidetracked by more interesting things

Silver
- Ignoring my body's signals that exercise is needed
- Inconvenience or too many decision points
- Getting sidetracked by more interesting things
- Lack of people to connect with during exercise

ACTIVITY

Bridging your barriers

The next step is to identify how these general barriers may appear in your life and ways you can avoid or overcome them. A great way to do this is to talk with another person. Here's how it works:

- First, pair off with someone of a similar color (your color or one of the colors closest to you on the color wheel)
- Then, spend two to three minutes jotting down your answers to the questions below
- After you've both completed writing, read your answers to each other, giving and getting feedback and ideas

1. Out of the possible barriers I identified from the barriers lists, the ONE most likely to challenge me as I increase or maintain my physical activity is …

2. This barrier will present itself in my life by …

(For example, if you chose the barrier of boredom, you might identify that you've tried to exercise in a gym with cardio machines, but you find that too hard to stick to because it's not entertaining or fun.)

3. How can I get around this barrier or overcome it quickly?

(List as many ideas as you want, as long as they are realistic and true to your color. Review your answers to the Put Your Preferences Into Practice activities on pages 21, 34, and 48 if needed)

Remember...

If you have more than one main barrier, you can repeat this exercise. Follow the three steps for identifying barriers and write down your answers.

Each of the five stages brings unique challenges and rewards, and trying to jump ahead or move through them too quickly can hurt your chances of long-term success. Remember, change is all about decision balance, increasing the pros and reducing the cons.

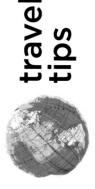

travel tips

Staying Active on the Road

We are on the move more than ever today, away from home on a regular basis for business and for pleasure. For many people, travel is part of life, not an exception, and we need be prepared so that we can take advantage of new workout opportunities and not get off track in different locations.

Blue

- Commit to yourself and schedule exercise as an appointment. Know your schedule ahead of time and plan exercise accordingly.
- Investigate gyms, swimming pools, and recreational paths. Know the hours of operation, rules, and pricing before you go.
- Keep it simple: choose familiar environments and familiar equipment.

Gold

- Commit to yourself and schedule exercise as an appointment. Know your schedule ahead of time and plan exercise accordingly.
- Develop an on-the-road plan with your trainer. Create a reporting system for accountability.
- Set goals that you can accomplish wherever you are, such as running three miles in every city you visit. Record and collect these accomplishments.

White

- Travel with your own personal training bag (resistance bands, a travel mat, etc.). With organization and advanced planning, you can have a full strength-training workout.
- Check out the hotel gym ahead of your workout and plan to exercise at off-peak times, away from colleagues.
- Take a hike! Get outside and enjoy nature, which can provide a calming effect after a busy day of interaction.

Purple

- Pack your comfortable shoes and check out walking distances ahead of time so you can accumulate exercise by walking to your appointments and meetings when possible.
- Find your way to the nearest gym and continue with your home fitness routine.
- Use travel as an opportunity to try something out of your routine — perhaps a different style of class.

Green

- Continue your training alone at the hotel or nearby gym if you're training for an event. Don't feel obligated to accept invitations from colleagues and fellow travelers inviting you to train together.
- Get outside. Nature trails, city parks, and bike paths are being built and maintained in most cities. Check out maps and websites for information.
- Climb high! Check out the highest peak wherever you are and go straight to the top. Savor the view at the highest elevation possible.

Red

- Find new friends and colleagues to play basketball or tennis with — before or after meetings.
- Build in an extra day or more for some action-packed recreation in the area when visiting a new part of the country or world.
- Train at the hotel or nearby gym — it's best to go when there are people around to have fun with and keep your energy up.

Saffron

- Keep your favorite music handy when traveling. It will keep you energized when walking or jogging in the park or on the treadmill.
- Get a boost of energy by exploring a city on foot. Taking in new sights, experiences, and local culture is primary. Exercise is secondary, but many miles and exercise are accomplished along the way.
- Be open to meeting colleagues for a walk or run when on the road. It's a great way to get exercise while conducting business.

Silver

- Just start walking and see where it takes you. What better way to explore a city than by foot? Walking can take you to new places, satisfying your natural curiosity.
- Suggest walking meetings prior to your arrival if possible. They're a great way to get exercise while conducting business.
- Keep moving. Go to your hotel or nearby gym dressed and ready to work out. Avoid anything that feels like a waste of time or has too many decision points.

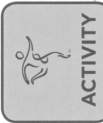

ACTIVITY

Creating a week-long program

Now that you're familiar with the preferences of your fitness personality, let's put them together with the CDC guidelines for physical activity. Refer to the Fitness Glossary in Chapter 3 and fill in the outline to create a four-day program.

Your Color:

150 minutes of moderate activity:

OR **75 minutes of vigorous activity in a week:**

Strength Training

"There is a vitality, a life force, an energy, a quickening, that is translated through you into action, and because there is only one of you in all time, this expression is unique."

-MARTHA GRAHAM

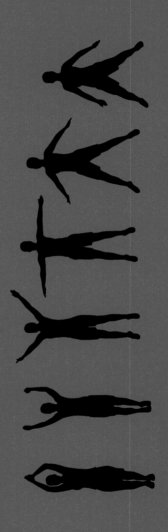

True Blue: Tried and True

Beat your barriers! See the top 10 tips

Common Barriers

- Not scheduling activity in advance
- Other responsibilities that could take priority
- Over-stimulating or dis-organized environments
- Disruption of routine or plan

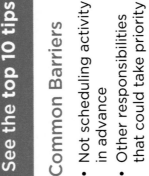

FACTOR 1

Motivators: Why do you exercise?

- Keeping the commitments I make to myself
- Finishing what I set out to do
- Having clear fitness goals
- Following advice from health professionals or trusted sources

FACTOR 2

Approach: How do you go about exercise?

- Choosing a proven program to accomplish my goals
- Being sensible and learning safe and correct exercise form from the start
- Building my program step-by-step and achieving measurable goals along the way
- Choosing a set exercise plan that I can make part of my routine

FACTOR 3

Focus: What engages your mind?

- Focusing on correct form and proper technique
- Concentrating on chanting, mantras, or songs
- Monitoring and measuring shorter- and longer-term exercise goals
- Reading or listening to audio recordings

FACTOR 4

Environment: Where do you most enjoy being physically active?

- Outdoor environments that are safe and predictable
- Familiar environments — same time, same place
- Fitness centers where I can get in and out quickly
- Larger gym environments where I can create my own space by using headphones or reading

FACTOR 5

Interpersonal Connections: Who do you exercise with?

- Find working out alone is energizing
- Prefer keeping exercise and socializing separate
- Focus on meeting my goals and avoid the distractions of others
- Might work out with a few others if goals can be achieved according to plan

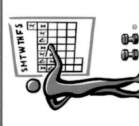

top 10 tips

1. Gather information from experts to establish the importance of physical activity.

2. Take steps to assure safety and avoid injury. Check equipment, and review techniques and routines with professionals.

3. Choose a gym or outdoor fitness site carefully, keeping in mind the need for calm and organization. Familiar paths and routes work best when exercising outdoors.

4. Make a commitment to yourself, which is a prime motivator for exercise.

5. Schedule exercise as an appointment and put it on the list.

6. When learning new routines, build slowly, ensuring correct technique at each stage.

7. Track progress and maintain records.

8. Keep exercise plans simple; make it easy to achieve your goals.

9. Use your powers of concentration to create your own environment. A smartphone and audiobooks can help you tune out distractions.

10. When traveling, investigate your fitness options ahead of time.

The Gold Standard: Just the Facts

FACTOR 1

Motivators: Why do you exercise?

- Keeping commitments to myself and others
- Sharing accomplishments with others
- Having clear fitness goals
- Following advice from health professionals or trusted sources

FACTOR 2

Approach: How do you go about exercise?

- Planning and scheduling my exercise program in advance
- Choosing a proven program to accomplish my goals
- Being responsible and learning safe and correct exercise form from the start
- Setting long-term goals, then breaking goals into smaller measurable pieces
- Choosing exercise I can make part of my routine

FACTOR 3

Focus: What engages your mind?

- Focusing on correct form and proper technique
- Concentrating on chanting, mantras, or songs
- Monitoring and measuring shorter- and longer-term exercise goals
- Listening to music or watching TV

FACTOR 4

Environment: Where do you most enjoy being physically active?

- Outdoor environments that are safe and predictable
- Familiar environments — same time, same place
- Fitness centers that are open and well lit
- Gyms with an organized and friendly atmosphere

FACTOR 5

Interpersonal Connections: Who do you exercise with?

- Enjoy having people in exercise environment, but not interacting directly
- Take pleasure in sharing accomplishments with others
- Are attracted to socializing around organized sporting activities
- Might work out with others as long as goals can be achieved according to plan

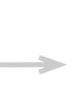

Beat your barriers! See the top 10 tips

Common Barriers

- Safety concerns
- Lacking clear goals for physical activity
- Not scheduling activity in advance
- Disruption of routine or plan

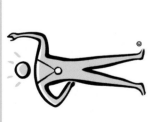

top 10 tips

1. Take steps to assure safety and avoid injury. Check equipment, and review techniques and routines with professionals.

2. Be clear about your purpose for physical activity and the benefits it can bring.

3. Choose activities that are proven and promise results.

4. Make a commitment to yourself and others.

5. Break larger goals down into smaller parts. Set a plan for each workout so you can enjoy the satisfaction of accomplishing it.

6. Aim to exercise at a consistent time when possible, keeping track of results.

7. Use physical activity as a time to reflect and think.

8. Enjoy accomplishing what you set out to do.

9. Interact with the outdoors.

10. Engage with activities that benefit the mind and body.

The White Canvas: Trailblazers on Familiar Paths

**Beat your barriers!
See the top 10 tips**

Common Barriers

- Not starting until the plan is fully in place
- Unfamiliar or jarring environments
- Disruption of routine or plan
- Lack of transition time to switch mental gears between activities

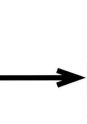

FACTOR 1

Motivators: Why do you exercise?

- Enjoying physical activities as a time to reflect and think
- Accomplishing what I set out to do
- Interacting with the outdoors
- Engaging with activities that benefit my mind and body

FACTOR 2

Approach: How do you go about exercise?

- Researching, then building a program based on my own vision and self-defined goals
- Planning my exercise program in advance
- Classifying exercise into types, such as cardio, strength, and flexibility
- Rotating these types throughout my exercise week
- Choosing exercise I can make part of my routine

FACTOR 3

Focus: What engages your mind?

- Attending to internal thoughts and letting things "pop up"
- Engaging in repetitive motion to zone out
- Enjoying familiar surroundings and predictable activities
- Reading or listening to audio recordings when engaged in routine cardio activities

FACTOR 4

Environment: Where do you most enjoy being physically active?

- Peaceful and calm environments
- Small, quiet, and uncrowded gyms
- Fitness centers that I have checked out prior to beginning my workout
- Outdoor environments with familiar paths and routes

FACTOR 5

Interpersonal Connections: Who do you exercise with?

- Reenergize by working out alone
- Enjoy peaceful, quiet settings
- Find unwanted chit-chat irritating
- Might work out with a few others as long as goals can be achieved according to plan

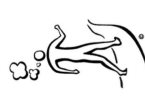

top 10 tips

1. Use your natural preference to organize into categories. Plan for cardio, stretching, and strength training.

2. Begin exercising, even without all the pieces in place.

3. Accept unfinished workouts as better than no workouts; commit to just 10 minutes and pick up where you left off next time.

4. Familiarize yourself with the fitness facility or environment before you actually go for a workout.

5. Carefully select environments that aren't distracting. Whenever possible, work out in calm and peaceful spaces.

6. Schedule solitary activities that provide balance to work, family, and other responsibilities.

7. Choose activities that are repetitive, providing refreshing and creative time alone.

8. Align with your desire for the familiar by choosing activities that you can make routine and fit into the rhythms of your life.

9. Your pace and interest in reflection make you especially sensitive to time pressure. Build buffer time on both sides of an activity to avoid feeling rushed.

10. Designate time to plan ahead for fitness activity on the road. Research resources and locations, and make a plan.

Royal Purple: Pursuers with a Plan

FACTOR 1 Motivators: Why do you exercise?

- Enjoying physical activities as a time to reflect and think
- Accomplishing what I set out to do
- Staying in shape and taking care of myself
- Finding balance in my life

FACTOR 2 Approach: How do you go about exercise?

- Researching and seeking information from others, then building a program based on my own vision and self-defined goals
- Planning my exercise program in advance
- Classifying exercise into types, such as cardio, strength, and flexibility
- Rotating these types throughout my exercise week
- Experimenting occasionally, but staying consistent by choosing exercise that can become part of my routine

FACTOR 3 Focus: What engages your mind?

- Attending to internal thoughts and letting things "pop up"
- Using repetitive motion as an opportunity to zone out
- Focusing on time, distance, or completing planned workout
- Reading, listening to audio recordings, or watching TV during routine cardio workouts

FACTOR 4 Environment: Where do you most enjoy being physically active?

- Outdoor environments with familiar paths and routes
- Any out-of-preference opportunity if it is convenient and offers a little variety in order to just do something
- Fitness centers with many choices of activity
- Gyms with an organized and friendly atmosphere

FACTOR 5 Interpersonal Connections: Who do you exercise with?

- Reenergize by working out alone
- Prefer to keep exercising and socializing separate
- Enjoy having other people in exercise environment, but not interacting directly
- Exercise near or alongside others for variety

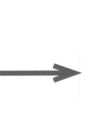

Beat your barriers!
See the top 10 tips

Common Barriers

- Trying to exercise without a plan
- Distracting or jarring environments
- Interruptions to my exercise plan
- Not making exercise a part of my lifestyle

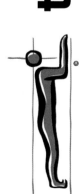

top 10 tips

1. Visualize, plan ahead, and schedule. You don't have to stick to your plan, but it's difficult to move forward without one.

2. Organize exercise into categories, for example: cardio, strength, flexibility; light, moderate, and intense; and indoor/outdoor.

3. Consult with a trainer to design a program for initial setup and knowledge; develop your own routine from there.

4. Choose an environment that's pleasing and supportive to physical exercise. Environments that feel unpleasant can negatively affect your workout.

5. Avoid being distracted by socializing during exercise. Purples tend to enjoy people in the environment, but not interacting directly with them. Save the socializing for later.

6. Align with your desire for the familiar by choosing activities that you can make routine and fit into the rhythms of your life.

7. Frame routine exercise as important alone/creative time.

8. Incorporate repetitious forms of exercise that do not require focused attention, allowing for your mind to relax.

9. Avoid exercise that requires navigational skills. Without comfortable landmarks, Purples can easily get lost, which creates anxiety and interferes with exercise.

10. Maintain interest by ensuring variety within a routine, and rotate throughout the week.

Greener than Green: Nature Beckons

FACTOR 1

Motivators: Why do you exercise?

- Reenergizing myself outdoors
- Having fun interacting with the outdoors
- Getting in shape for meaningful outdoor activities
- Increasing my self reliance and preparedness

FACTOR 2

Approach: How do you go about exercise?

- Keeping gear handy to be ready for action
- Staying open to unplanned physical activity
- Connecting with my playful personality while avoiding joyless exercise that feels never-ending
- Putting exercise into daily living activities
- Having easy access to the outdoors

FACTOR 3

Focus: What engages your mind?

- Using outstanding direction and observation skills
- Taking in the physical surroundings, including smells and sounds
- Responding to activities and actions
- Noticing details in nature

FACTOR 4

Environment: Where do you most enjoy being physically active?

- Outdoors in nature
- Gyms if in preparation for an important outdoor event
- Anywhere I can have fun using my outstanding navigational skills
- The highest point for the best scenery and views, wherever I am

FACTOR 5

Interpersonal Connections: Who do you exercise with?

- Enjoy being alone in nature
- Exercise alone to enable flexibility and quick response
- Prefer training for a goal without others
- Compete with others to inspire better performance and have fun

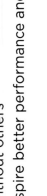

Beat your barriers! See the **top 10 tips**

Common Barriers

- Boredom of routine exercise
- Not getting outside into nature
- Missing chances to include activity in my daily living
- Difficulty finding time alone to exercise

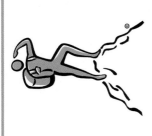

top 10 tips

1. Create time to be outdoors alone. Negotiate work and family responsibilities to ensure that time.

2. Investigate nature preserves, recreational paths, and waterways near work and home. The great outdoors might be closer than you think.

3. Find natural and convenient ways to include exercise in the activities of daily living — yard work, stone work, housework, walking to destinations, and using stairs instead of elevators.

4. Combine activity with productivity and contributing to your community. For example, work on building a nature trail or help maintain the grounds at a park.

5. Share your love of the outdoors with children. Lead a scouting troop, coach a team, or play outside with children. Think about teaching a nature class.

6. Train for an outdoor challenge or meaningful activity by yourself. Don't be pressured into being an exercise buddy.

7. Enjoy nature in all its forms and at all times of day. Don't rule out nighttime; it provides one more opportunity with another set of sensations.

8. With your love of vistas and views, make sure you go to the top. That's what makes it worth the climb.

9. Revisit favorite places. Enjoy noticing physical changes, both big and small.

10. Bring your binoculars, camera, or compass — these items make your time outside even more fun and fascinating.

Roaring Reds: Now!

FACTOR 1

Motivators: Why do you exercise?

- Reenergizing myself outdoors
- Having fun interacting with the outdoors
- Enjoying a physically active lifestyle
- Engaging in fun competitive activities with others

FACTOR 2

Approach: How do you go about exercise?

- Seeking activities that I find fun, yet challenging
- Participating in activities that are personally appealing and often unusual
- Connecting with my playful personality while avoiding joyless exercise
- Choosing activities that are convenient, requiring very little process and advanced planning
- Having fun with many types of exercise

FACTOR 3

Focus: What engages your mind?

- Taking in the physical surroundings, including smells and sounds
- Responding to activities and actions
- Having a goal to provide focus and relieve exercise boredom
- Listening to energetic music or watching action TV during cardio workouts at the gym

FACTOR 4

Environment: Where do you most enjoy being physically active?

- Outdoors in nature
- Anywhere high energy and action packed
- Well-lit gyms offering cardio equipment with a view
- At home, with fitness equipment where it can be seen

FACTOR 5

Interpersonal Connections: Who do you exercise with?

- Keep the momentum going by interacting with others
- Treat physical activity with others as a way of life
- Prefer training for a goal with others
- Compete with others to inspire better performance and have fun

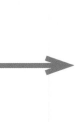

Beat your barriers! See the top 10 tips

Common Barriers

- Boredom of routine exercise
- Lack of people to connect with during exercise
- Not having a goal
- Not getting outdoors

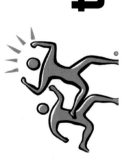

top 10 tips

1. You are likely to be bored by pure exercise. Stay in shape by choosing activities and sports that are fun and can be done with others. Maintain a network of active people you can enjoy physical activity and sports with.

2. Train for an event with others. The event provides motivation and energy for peak performance, and training with others makes it fun.

3. Keep your smartphone handy and filled with your favorite music to keep you moving, especially when exercising inside.

4. Avoid making commitments that may get in the way of your freedom and flexibility. Over scheduling can be a turnoff.

5. Maintain momentum by keeping your goals in sight. Post notes, action pictures, and other reminders of what you want to achieve.

6. Keep gear handy so you will be ready for action when an opportunity opens up.

7. To avoid injury, resist your natural impulse to overdo it every time. Go easy on yourself when recovering from an injury or getting back in shape.

8. Create mini goals along the way, such as time, distance, or improvement.

9. Get outside. With your outstanding observation and navigation skills, you won't be bored in outdoor settings.

10. If you use indoor equipment, find or move it near a window so you can enjoy views of nature and outdoor activity.

Saffrons Seeking: Making Workouts into Play

Beat your barriers!
See the top 10 tips

Common Barriers

- Ignoring my body's signals that exercise is needed
- Not valuing the importance of fun activity
- Inconvenience or too many decision points
- Getting sidetracked by more interesting things

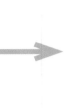

 FACTOR 1

Motivators: Why do you exercise?

- Reducing internal stress and boosting energy
- Finding pleasure in difficult, interesting, and unusual challenges
- Participating in activities that benefit my mind and body
- Seeking enjoyment in the activity, with exercise as an added benefit

 FACTOR 2

Approach: How do you go about exercise?

- Seeking activities that I find fun, yet challenging
- Participating in activities that are personally appealing and often unusual
- Connecting with my playful personality while avoiding joyless exercise
- Choosing activities that are convenient, requiring very little process and advanced planning

 FACTOR 3

Focus: What engages your mind?

- Listening to music while active
- Having a challenge or a goal to focus on
- Directing attention on an activity while getting exercise along the way
- Having fun because exercise is boring by itself

 FACTOR 4

Environment: Where do you most enjoy being physically active?

- Outdoors in natural surroundings and fresh air
- Somewhere easily accessible with few barriers to getting started
- Outdoors when doing cardio activities
- Fitness centers with a casual atmosphere and dress code

 FACTOR 5

Interpersonal Connections: Who do you exercise with?

- Are attracted to independent activities alongside other people
- Enjoy activities with others that are easily coordinated and fun
- Keep momentum high by light conversation with others
- Think and plan while they exercise alone

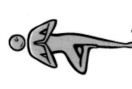

top 10 tips

1. Notice the physical signs of inactivity, such as aches, pains, stiffness, or soreness. Remember that getting more activity will help relieve these symptoms.

2. Anything that seems like pure exercise is boring and difficult to sustain. Choose activities that allow you to focus on something else and get exercise along the way.

3. Engage your fun/playful side. Avoid structured activities with rigid attendance requirements.

4. To keep your energy up, download your favorite music on your smart-phone and take it with you when walking or running.

5. Do your aerobic activities outdoors as much as possible.

6. Identify multiple locations for variety and spontaneity, including environments near home and work.

7. If you train in a gym, shop for the right gym, where you'll feel like yourself and where you're able to exercise as you choose and dress to be comfortable.

8. Enjoy solitary activities alongside others. With a comfortable person, light banter can provide just the right amount of engagement to spark your energy.

9. Respond to your desire for flow. Keep your gear handy and in ready-to-go condition so you can be your spontaneous self.

10. Choose activities and environments that engage you enough to quiet your internal critic.

Quicksilver: Masters of Exercise Disguise

FACTOR 1

Motivators: Why do you exercise?

- Responding to threats to health and well-being
- Finding pleasure in exploration and novel experiences
- Participating in activities that benefit my mind and body
- Seeking enjoyment in the activity, with exercise as an added benefit

FACTOR 2

Approach: How do you go about exercise?

- Participating in activities that hold my attention with many layers of achievement and interest
- Connecting with my playful personality while avoiding joyless exercise
- Choosing activities that are convenient, requiring very little process and advanced planning
- Keeping exercise simple and easy to complete

FACTOR 3

Focus: What engages your mind?

- Learning something new and interesting
- Having a challenge or a goal to focus on
- Directing attention on an activity while getting exercise along the way
- Focusing on the mind-body connection

FACTOR 4

Environment: Where do you most enjoy being physically active?

- Outdoors in natural surroundings and fresh air
- Somewhere easily accessible with few barriers to getting started
- Anywhere that offers many choices of activities and times
- New environments where I can explore and get exercise along the way

FACTOR 5

Interpersonal Connections: Who do you exercise with?

- Coordinate exercise with others to create accountability
- Include others in physical activity to make it fun and help pass the time
- Think and plan while they exercise alone

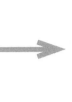

**Beat your barriers!
See the top 10 tips**

Common Barriers

- Ignoring my body's signals that exercise is needed
- Inconvenience or too many decision points
- Getting sidetracked by more interesting things
- Lack of people to connect with during exercise

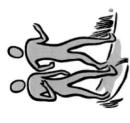

top 10 tips

1. Notice the physical signs of inactivity, such as aches, pains, stiffness, or soreness. Getting more activity will help relieve these symptoms.

2. Just begin your activity and see where it takes you. Don't wait until you can do it at the highest level or until conditions are otherwise perfect. Once you start working out, you're more likely to continue.

3. It's not about exercise. Disguise activity within something more appealing than exercise — make it part of something that's enjoyable and engaging.

4. Train for an event, which is a great way to spend time with other people, beat the boredom, and focus your interests.

5. Keep transitions minimal and decision points few. Don't get sidetracked along the way. For example, go to the gym in workout clothes to avoid wasted time in the locker room.

6. Convenience is a priority. Choose activities that can be easily accessed and keep equipment and workout gear handy.

7. Look for activities that are fun and can be easily slipped into the day.

8. Choose activities that will provide an opportunity to explore and learn something new.

9. Identify multiple locations for variety and freedom of choice, including environments near home and work.

10. Be accountable to others to combat the "do I feel like it?" threat to your activities. Working out with others is fun and raises your performance level.

NOTES

Use this page to reflect on what you've learned, both about The 8 Colors program and about yourself.

Consider the following questions as a guide:

What have been your key takeaways during this program?

What stage are you in now? What stage were you in at the beginning of the program?

Will you make any changes as a result of this program? Describe.

Additional comments...

be well!

BIBLIOGRAPHY

Beck, Martha. *The Four-Day Win: End Your Diet War and Achieve Thinner Peace.* New York: Rodale, 2008. Print.

Brue, Suzanne. *The 8 Colors of Fitness: Discover Your Color-Coded Fitness Personality and Create an Exercise Program You'll Never Quit!* Delray Beach: Oakledge Press, 2008. Print.

Moore, Margaret, and Bob Tschannen-Moran. *Coaching Psychology Manual,* Baltimore: Lippincot-Wolters, 2010. Print.

Prochaska, James O., John C. Norcross, and Carlo C. DiClemente *Changing For Good: A Revolutionary Six-Stage Program for Overcoming Bad Habits and Moving Your Life Positively Forward.* New York: Morrow-Harper, 1995. Print.

United States. Dept. of Health and Human Services. Centers for Disease Control and Prevention. *2008 Physical Activity Guidelines for Americans: Be Active, Healthy, and Happy.* By Janet E. Fulton and Howard W. Kohl. Oct. 2008. Web.

© 2015 by Suzanne Brue
Published by Oakledge Press, Delray Beach, Florida

ISBN-13: 978-0-9795625-1-8

Made in the USA
Monee, IL
24 June 2021